Northern Style

Siu Wan Kuen

Small Circular Fist

Rick L. Wing

Jing Mo Athletic Association

San Francisco, California

First Printing

Published by
Jing Mo Association
San Francisco, California
www.jingmo.com

ISBN 978-1688259782

Disclaimer

Please note that the author and publisher of this book are not responsible in any manner whatsoever for any injury that may result from practicing the techniques and/or following the instructions given in this book. Since the physical activities described may be too strenuous in nature to engage in safely, it is essential that a physician be consulted prior to training.

Dedicated to Grandmaster Ma Kin Fung

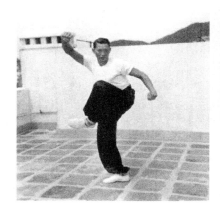
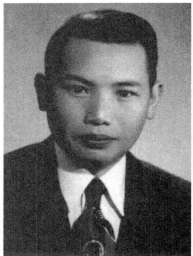
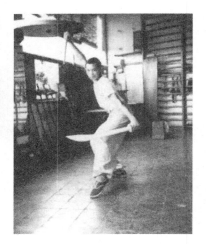
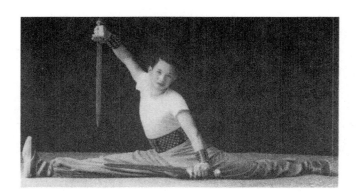

and

Sifu Danny S. Y. Ma (Ma Shun Yin), son of Ma Kin Fung.

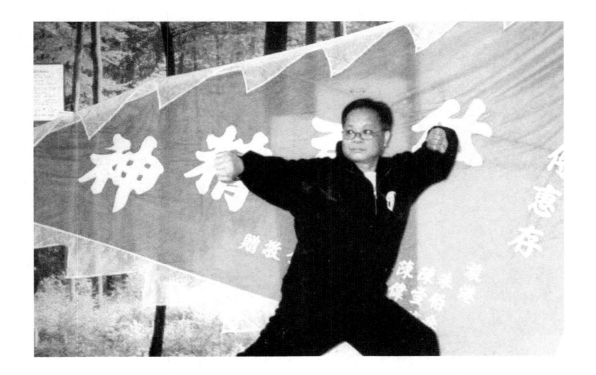

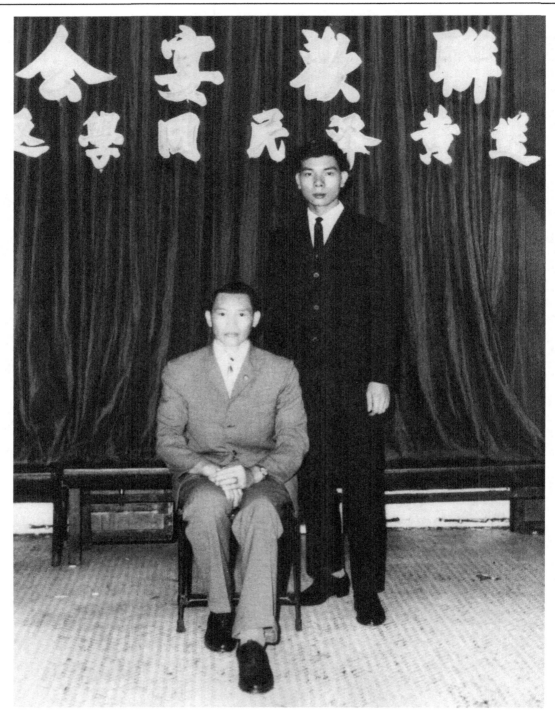

Wong Jack Man (standing, right) with Ma Kin Fung (sitting, left)

Calligraphy from Sifu Danny Ma to Rick L. Wing

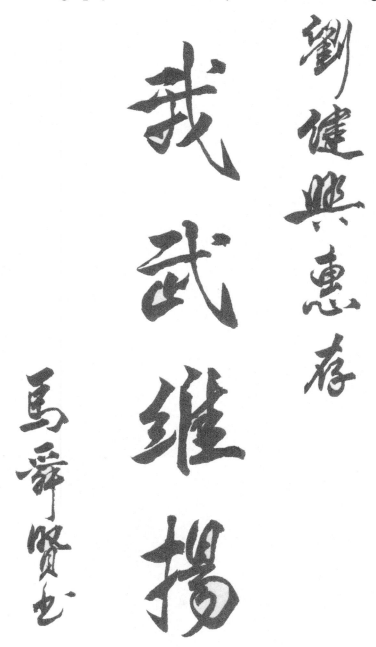

Low Gin Hing (Rick L. Wing), For Memory,
May our martial arts continue to grow and propagate widely.
Written by Ma Shun Yin (Sifu Danny S Y. Ma)

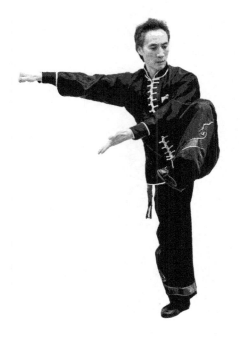

Contents

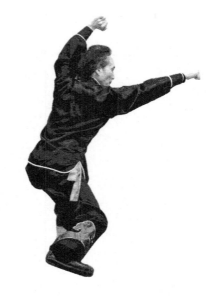

Preface

As I get older, I feel the need to have books to supplement my teaching of kung fu because... well, it's getting harder for me to do the moves over and over (and over) again. I can show the moves to my (few) students a few times, but I am of the age now where I simply cannot do the moves an indeterminate number of times. In addition to my aging and weakening physique, my patience also wears thin, so I wish to have a back-up – in other words, this book. Perhaps one day when I'm feeling lazy, I will just say, "Ah, look at my book, and go up to movement #8 today." Perhaps I won't even need to do the moves at all. Perhaps I will point and turn the pages. Better yet, maybe I can make a video or on-line course out of it so I won't need to show up at all! My limit is now just three or four times, and I am evolving to teach the way my teacher taught; this way I won't tire myself out. Maybe it is a blessing not to have so many students. I was also inspired to do this book for my friends in Germany who follow Grandmaster Al Dacascos, founder of the Wun Hop Kuen Do (WHKD) system of martial arts. Personally, I think there are more people *there* who practice Siu Wan Kuen than *here*. Who could possibly have imagined that?

The original intention of my series of books was to document the Northern Shaolin Style as taught by Sifu Wong Jack Man. I believe it may also be useful to document some of the basic sets he taught. Perhaps these books on the basic sets will have an even wider audience as more people learn the basic forms than the advanced forms. I consider Siu Wan Kuen to be a hidden gem of our kung fu heritage, and I offer my greatest respect to Grandmaster Ma Kin Fung for creating it. This is definitely one of my favorite sets to practice and demonstrate. And, if I forget this set, there is always this book!

Rick L. Wing
Fourth of July, 2019
Year of the Earth Pig, 4717
San Francisco, California

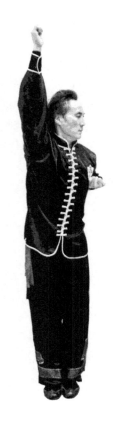

Commentary on Siu Wan Kuen

Siu Wan Kuen translates to "small circular fist." There are circular moves in this set, but then, there are circular moves in almost every kung fu set. Perhaps the name is inspired by the circular hand movements near the beginning of the set. Or perhaps the name is inspired by the circular and arcing moves throughout the set.

Most kung fu sets have origins that are shrouded in mystery, but the origin of this set is well known. This set was created from the experience and genius of Master Ma Kin Fung (Ma Gim Fung in Cantonese, or Ma-Sword-Wind). It was patterned after the well-known set "Gung Lick Kuen" (Gong Li Quan in pinyin) which means "to work one's strength." If one knows or has seen Gung Lick, the similarities are clear, especially in the early part of the form. Personally, I like this set better than Gung Lick Kuen. In my opinion it is more dynamic, the moves flow better, and I like these techniques more. Gung Lick seems to have the flavor of a drill-type form, as opposed to Siu Wan Kuen's more "expressive" and natural techniques. Gung Lick also has fewer kicking techniques, just two, and its emphasis seems to be more on hand techniques and low horse stances. Of course, this is my opinion and who am I to argue or debate with the thousands of people who know, practice and love Gung Lick Kuen.

Although this set is typically taught to beginners, it is much more than that, and advanced practitioners could spend a lifetime mastering these techniques. The set has left and right front heel kicks, a right front toe kick, left and right side kicks, and a sweeping hook kick. There are no jumping kicks, unusual for a northern set but very typical for a beginner's set. There are double punches, arm-breaks, basic blocks, vertical and horizontal fist strikes, chops, elbow strikes, claps and palm thrusts.

When doing this set, one must also twist and turn as if fighting multiple opponents. Some of the kicks may be done with full-extension to stretch the ligaments and tendons. Kicking high for practice and low for practical self-defense is the norm in northern styles. The hand strikes may also be done for the purpose of application or to enhance health by stretching out one's body. Notice that some of the kicks and strikes are extended to the sky so as to stretch and strengthen the arms and back. Notice the technique in the beginning where both palms are thrust upward, thus exercising the arms and the back. In the middle section of the set, after standing up from a crouch, a single right fist is also thrust skyward. In northern styles especially, many of the moves are for exercise and may not mimic the application exactly.

The postures and movements of the set stretch and extend the body. This is good for the spine and the body's carriage. Practicing with the body hunched over is not a northern characteristic.

Personally, I enjoy demonstrating this set in kung fu exhibitions as it flows well, has the overall feel of a northern style, and is not too taxing to the body; in other words, it's short, and I like that.

I've also created my own descriptive names for the movements and I hope this helps people remember the set more easily. (Note: It was actually Wong Jack Man who described movement #11 as "Double dragon fists.")

Students of Ma Kin Fung, such as my instructor, Wong Jack Man, teach this set as part of their curriculum. There are many others who teach this set since Ma had many disciples, some of whom went to Australia, Canada, New Zealand, Brazil and the United States of America and if more people incorporate this set into their curriculum, perhaps one day, Siu Wan Kuen will become as well-known as Gung Lick Kuen!

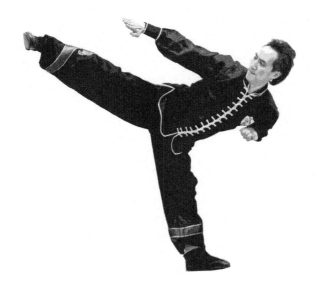

SIU WAN KUEN - THE FORM

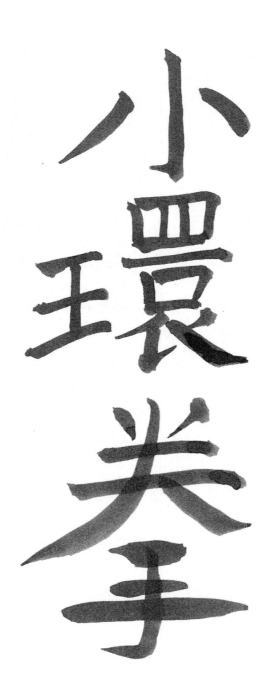

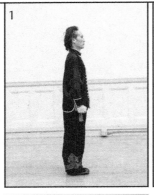

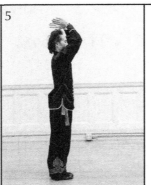

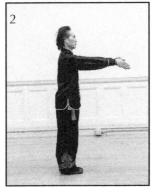

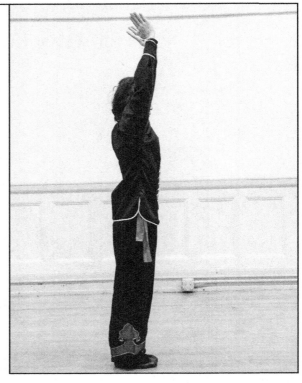

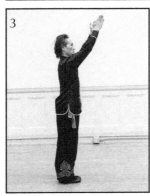

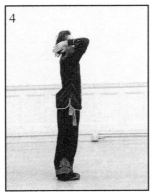

1. Listen for Buddha, Thrust palms to the sky.

Stand at attention. Bend the elbows and raise the hands to the ears. Bring both hands forward, then back and upwards so that both palms face inward.

Thrust both hands upwards with the blade edge of both palms facing up.

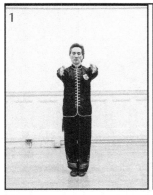

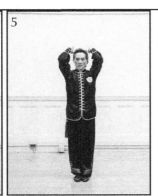

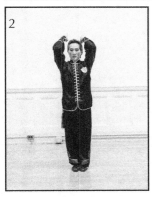

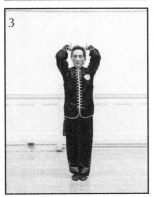

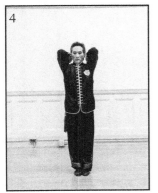

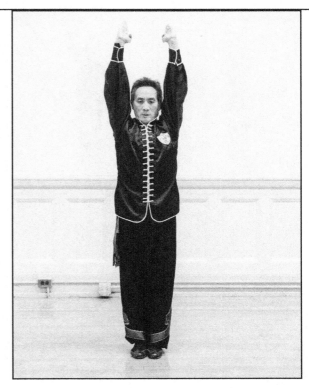

1. (Side view)

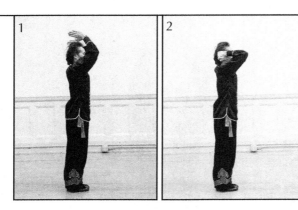

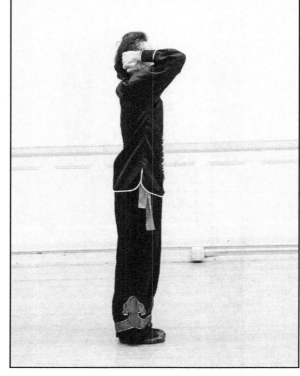

2. Pull hands down to the ears and form fists with both hands.

Pull hands down to the ears and form fists with both hands. Bring both hands down strongly and form fists.

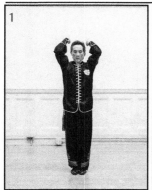
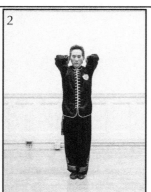

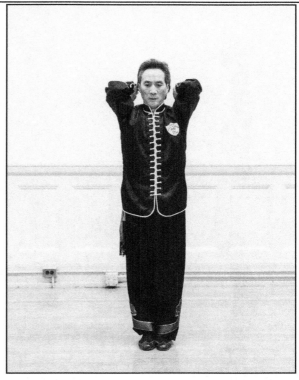

2. (Side view)

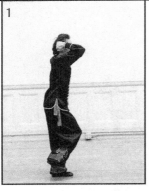

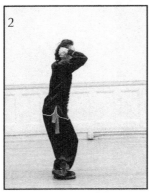

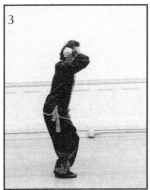

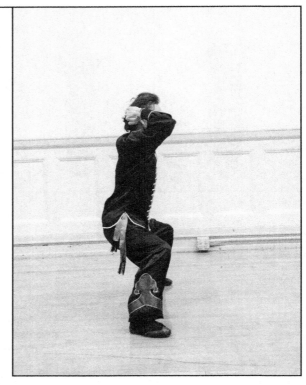

3. Stamp the right foot. Horse stance.

Stamp the right foot. Step the left foot to the left and sit in a horse stance. Step out into a horse stance by stepping the left foot to your left side.

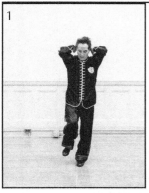

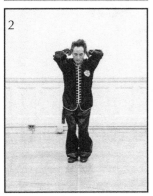

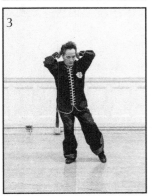

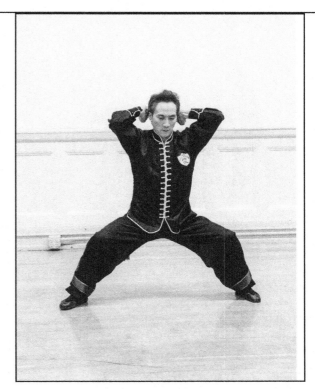

3. (Side view)

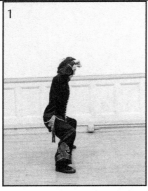

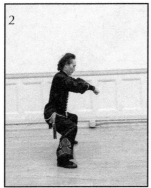

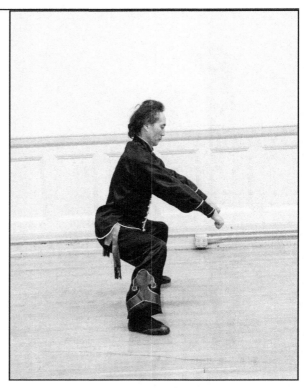

4. Double fists strike downward.

Double fists strike downward. Strike downward with horizontal fists. Your arms will be approximately at a 30 to 45 degree angle to your torso.

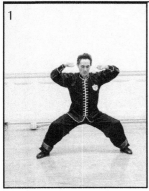

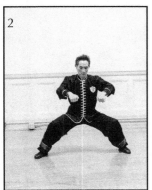

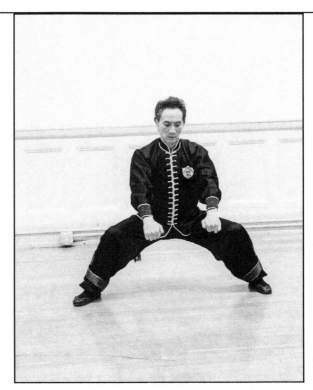

4. (Side view)

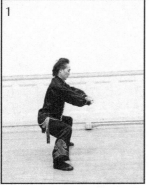

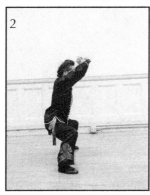

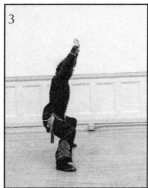

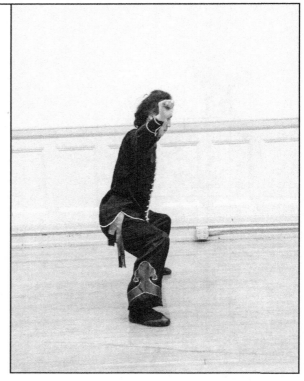

5. "X" (Cross) block above the head.

"X" (Cross) block above the head. Left forearm on top, right forearm on bottom. Raise both arms up and outward.

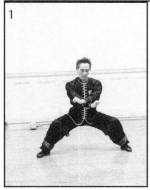

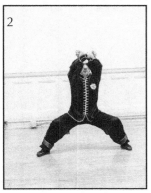

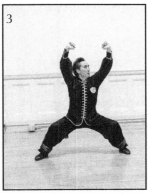

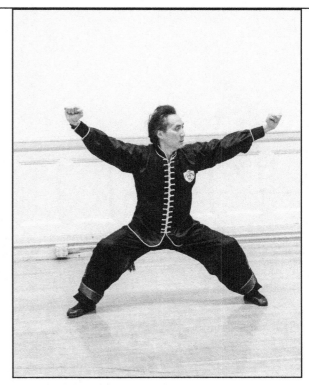

5. (Side view)

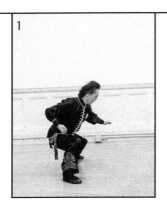

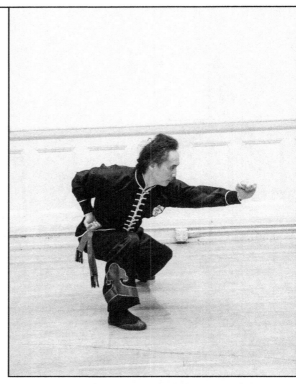

6. Left punch. Twisted stance.

Left punch (counterclockwise) to the right side. Twisted stance. Left knee forward. Continuing the circular motion of the arms, strike with a left vertical fist to your right side. As you twist your stance to the right, the right foot is on the flat of the foot and the left foot is on the ball of the foot.

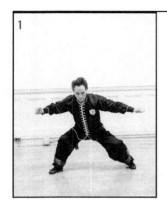

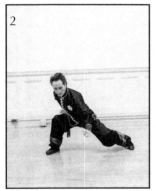

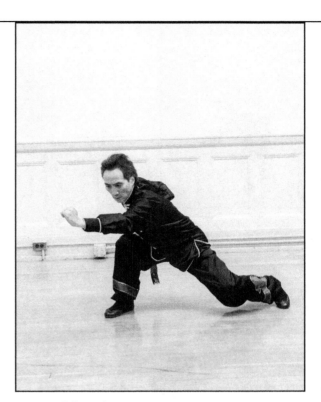

6. (Side view)

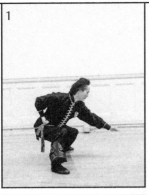

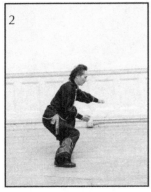

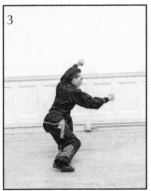

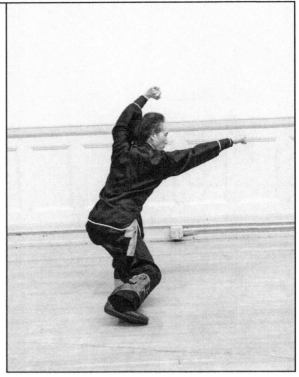

7. Right punch. Strike straight ahead. Twisted stance. Right knee forward.

Block down clockwise with the left fist. Uppercut strike (clockwise) with the right fist. Strike straight ahead. Twisted stance. Right knee forward.

Block down and then upward with the left forearm and then strike directly forward with a right horizontal fist. You may keep your right arm bent or extend it forward. Either way is acceptable. The left foot is now on the flat of the foot and the right foot is on the ball of the foot.

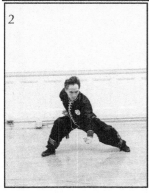

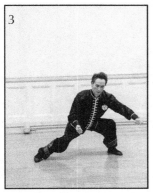

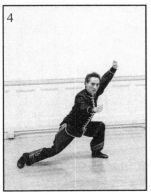

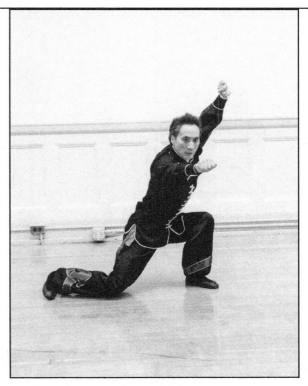

7. (Side view)

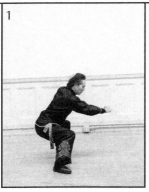

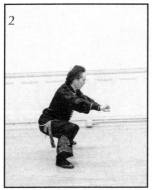

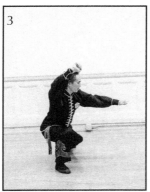

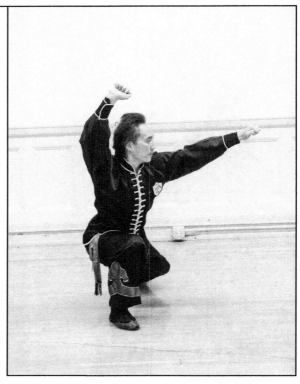

8. Left punch. Strike straight ahead. Twisted stance. Left knee forward.

Block down (counterclockwise) with the right fist. Uppercut strike with the left fist. Strike straight ahead. Twisted stance. Left knee forward.

Block down and then upward with the right forearm and then strike directly forward with a left horizontal fist. You may keep your left arm bent or extend it forward. Either way is acceptable. The right foot is now on the flat of the foot and the left foot is on the ball of the foot.

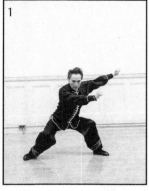

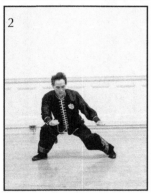

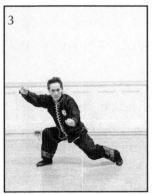

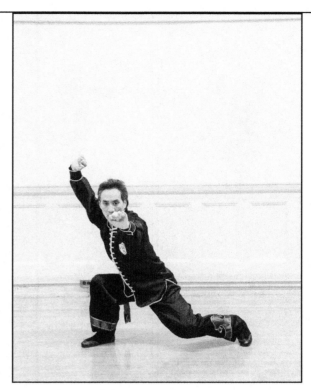

8. (Side view)

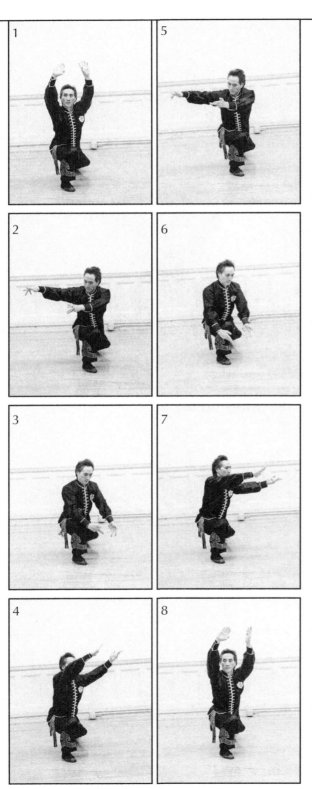

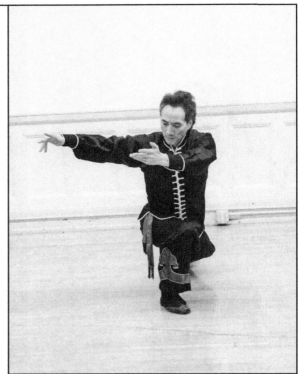

9) Double (clockwise) circular hands. Three times. Move hands like the wind. Create a whirlwind with the hands.

Twist your squatting stance slightly to the right and make three (or two) large clockwise circular motions with both of your hands. At the top of the circle, the palms will face outward but at the lower part of the circle, the palms will face inward (towards you). Move your arms continuously. Remember that kung fu forms are to flow from one movement to another.

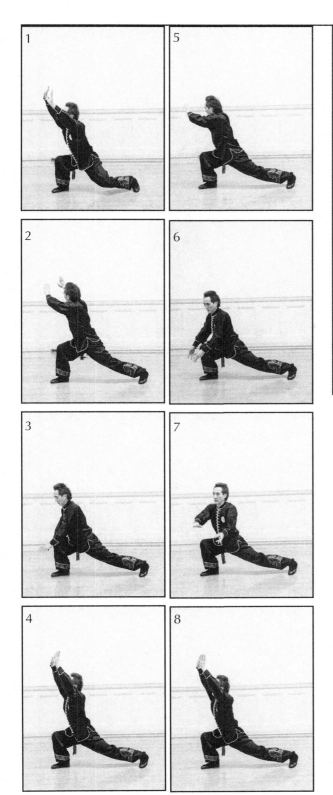

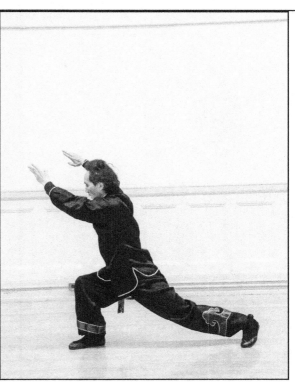

9. (Side view)

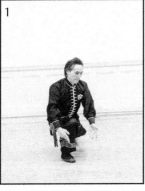

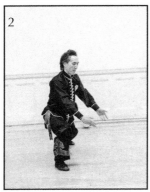

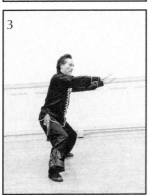

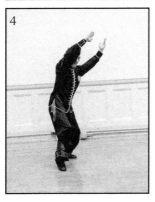

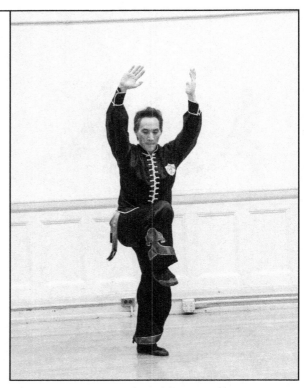

10. Raise the right leg. Raise both hands high.

Raise the right leg. Right instep flexed upward. Raise both hands high. After the last circle and as the hands are rising up, lift the right leg and bend it at the knee. As the foot is being raised, flex the right instep upward. Movement #11 immediately follows from movement #10 and the hands never stop moving until movement #11 is completed.

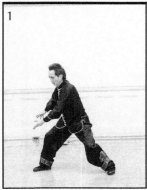

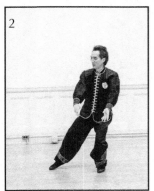

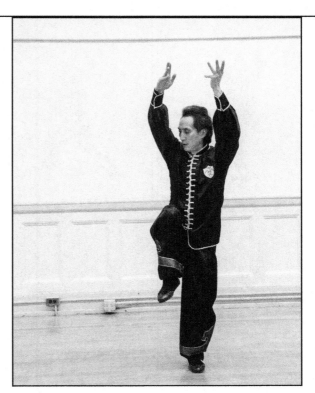

10. (Side view)

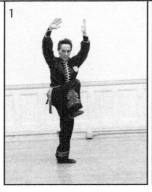

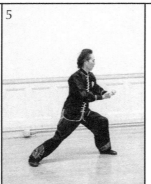

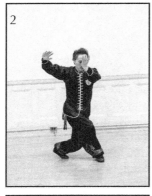

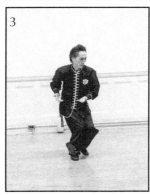

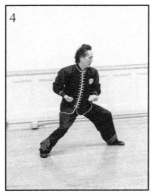

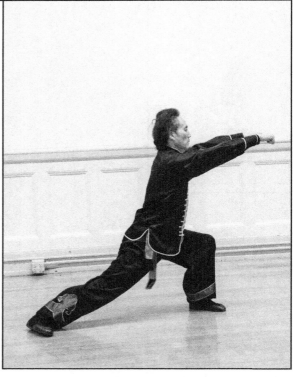

11. Double dragons (horizontal) fist strike. Double charging fists. Clockwise motion. Left bow stance.

Continuing the clockwise motion of the arms, step down with the right foot past the left foot and step into a left bow stance. Strike hard with double horizontal fists.

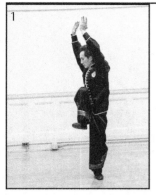

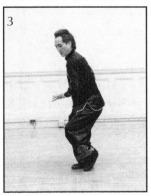

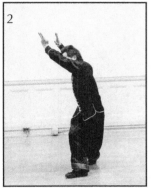

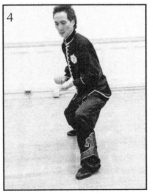

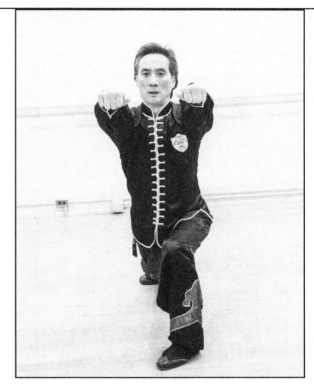

11. (Side view)

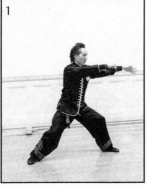

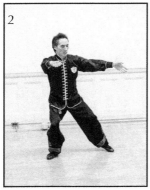

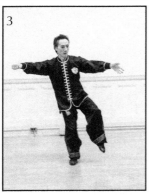

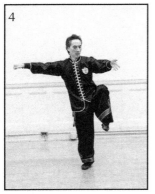

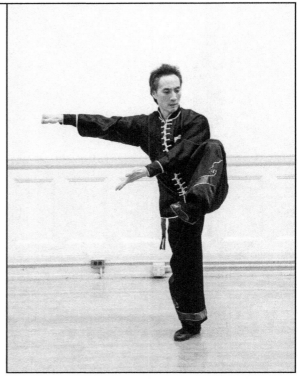

12. Step back. Crane stance. Left leg raised. Left palm faces the sky.

Swing the right arm backward in a clockwise arc and form a fist with the right hand. Following this motion, swing the left arm backward, also in a clockwise arc, and open the left hand.

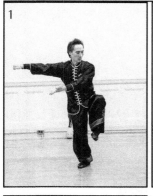

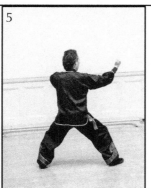

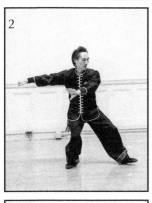

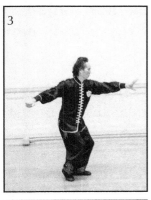

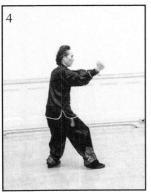

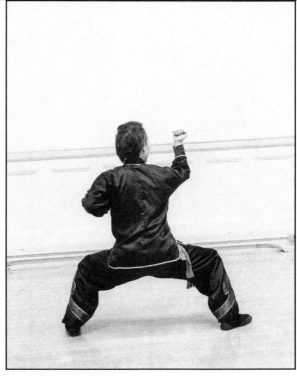

13. Left grabbing hand. Left foot steps down into a horse stance. Right arm (forearm or fist) breaks the opponent's arm.

Step down with the left foot and bring the right foot past the left. Sit in a horse stance. At the same time, make a counterclockwise grabbing motion with the left hand. Strike sideways with the right forearm and clench the right hand into a fist.

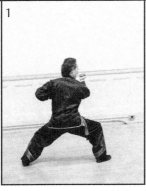

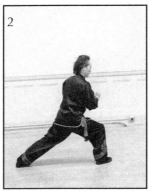

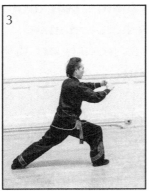

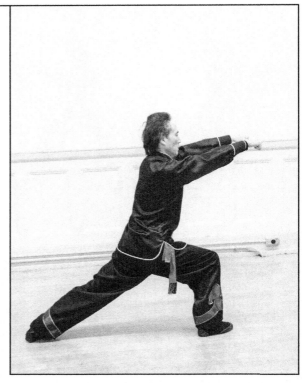

14. Double dragon (horizontal) fists. Strike to the right. Right bow stance.

Shift your horse into a right bow stance. Strike to your right with double horizontal fists. Your right fist moves in a slight counterclockwise arc rearward and then forward while the left fist shoots forward straight to the right.

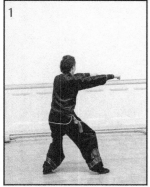

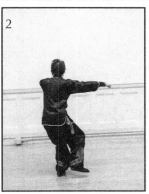

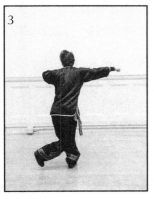

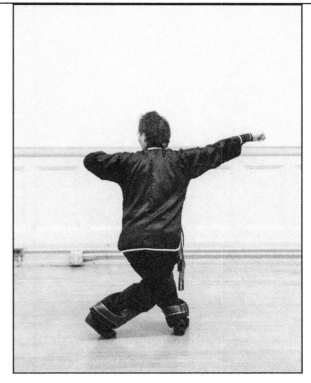

15. Step back into left T-stance. Left battering elbow strike.

Step the right foot behind the left leg into a left T-stance. Strike with the left elbow.

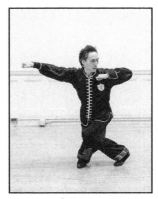

Back View

45

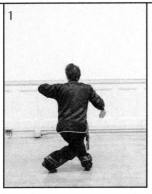

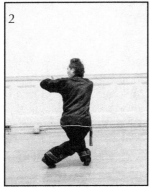

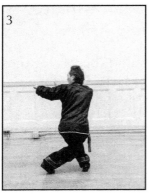

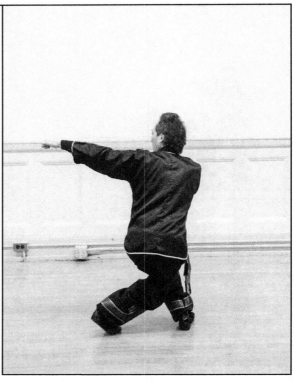

16. Right hand to the guard position. Left (horizontal) punch.

Bring the right hand down and to the left and open the right palm alongside the left fist. Then strike to your left with a left horizontal fist.

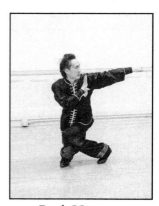

Back View

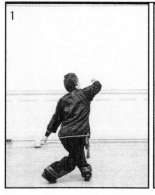

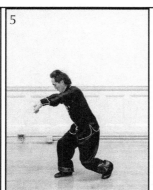

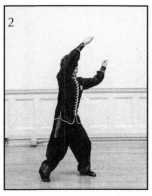

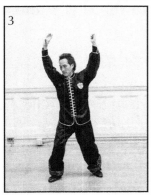

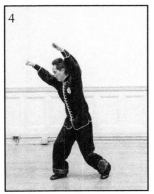

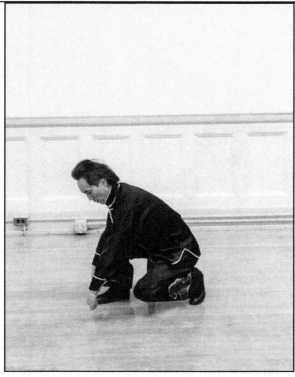

17. Turn to the right. Reach to the sky. Right grabbing hand. Left fist follows. Smash down to the ground. Crouching stance.

Turn to your right and make a large clockwise motion with the right hand. The right hand will open and then close into a right fist. The left fist will follow the right hand and then both hands will come down as fists. The legs will rise up and then fall down into the crouching stance. The flat of the right foot is on the ground and the ball of the left foot is on the ground.

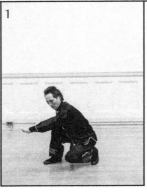

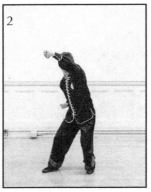

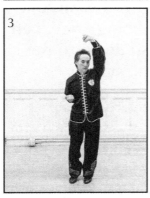

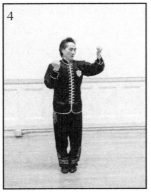

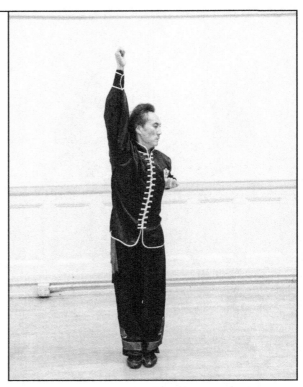

18. Right punch to the sky. Stand up straight.

Turn 90 degrees to the left. The left foot moves slightly to the left and the right foot will move to the left to be alongside the right side of the left foot. Make a counterclockwise clearing block with the left forearm and strike directly upward with the right vertical fist. Stand up straight.

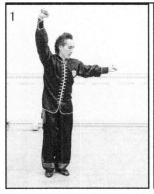

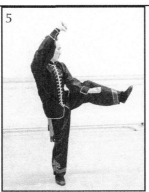

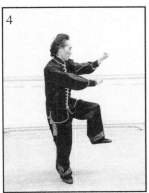

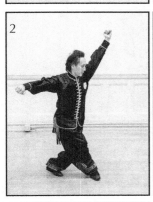

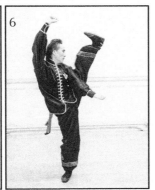

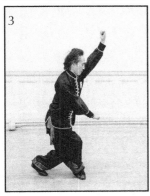

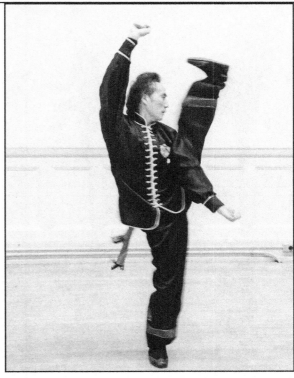

19. Right hand blocks up. Left backfist strikes down. Left heel kick.

Turn to your left side and move the right arm down in a clockwise motion. At the same time, lift the left arm upward in a clockwise motion. Step the right foot past the left into a right T-stance. While blocking upward with the right hand, strike down with a left backfist. At the same time, kick up with a high left heel kick.

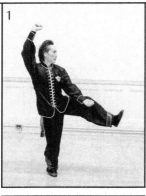

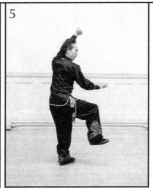

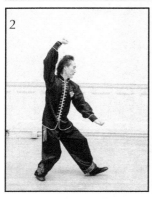

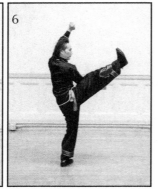

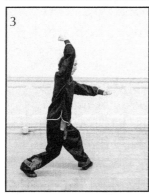

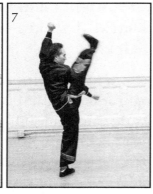

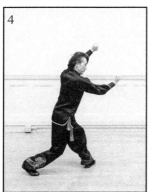

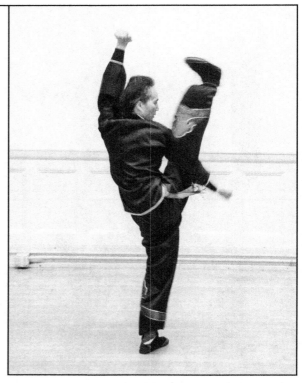

20. Left hand blocks up. Right backfist strikes down. Right heel kick.

Put the left foot down and do a similar motion except it is on the other side. Block upward with the left hand, strike down with the right, and kick upward with a high right heel kick.

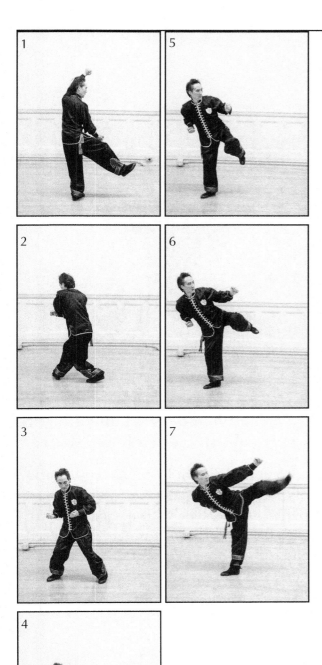

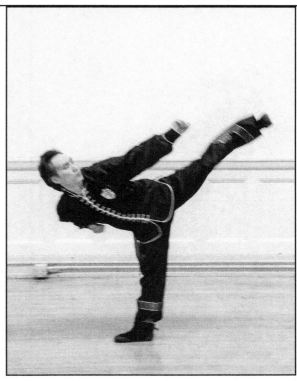

21. Turn around. Left side kick. Left vertical punch.

Turn to your left and bring the right foot past the front of the left leg. You will temporarily sit in a right T-stance. Then continue turning to your left and cross your forearms (left over the right) and bring both fists back to the side of your body. The weight is now on the right leg. Lift the left leg and as you kick out with a left side kick, strike outward at about face level using a left vertical fist.

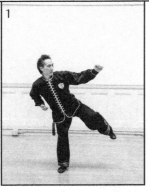

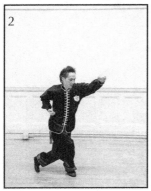

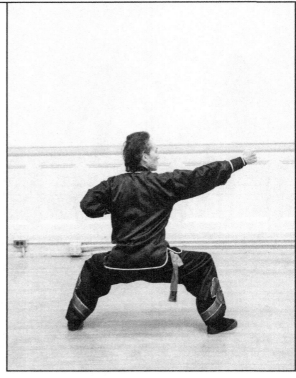

22) Left hand blocks down. Right vertical fist. Sit in a horse stance.

Bring the left foot back, passing in back of the right leg. Momentarily, sit into a right T-stance. Block down (clockwise) with the left forearm. Turn your to the left and strike with a right vertical fist. Sit in a horse stance.

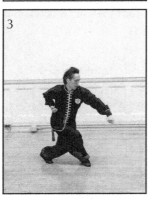

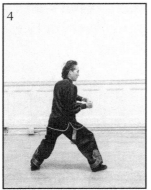

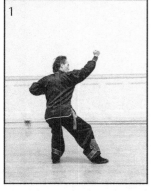

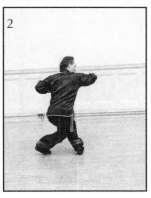

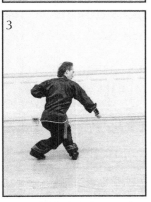

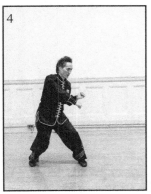

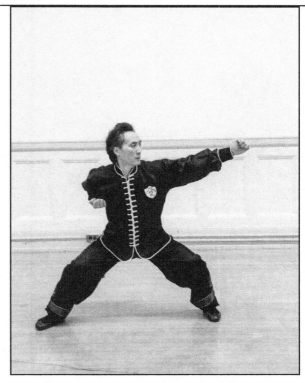

23) Right hand blocks down. Left vertical fist. Sit in a horse stance.

Step back with the right leg. Momentarily sitting in a left T-stance. Block down (counterclockwise) with the right forearm. Turn to the right and strike with a left vertical fist. Sit in a horse stance.

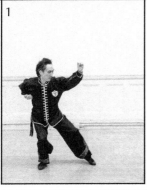

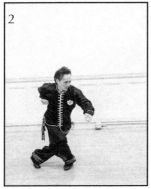

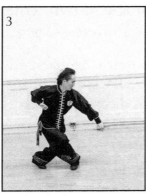

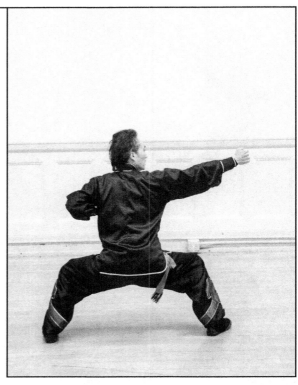

24) Left hand blocks down. Right vertical fist. Sit in a horse stance.

Bring the left foot back, passing in back of the right leg. Momentarily, sit into a right T-stance. Block down (clockwise) with the left forearm. Turn to the left and strike with a right vertical fist. Sit in a horse stance.

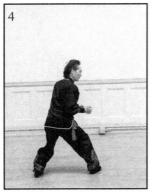

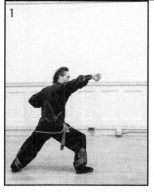

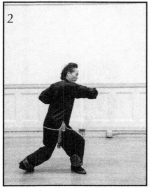

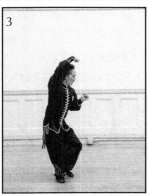

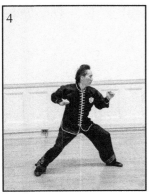

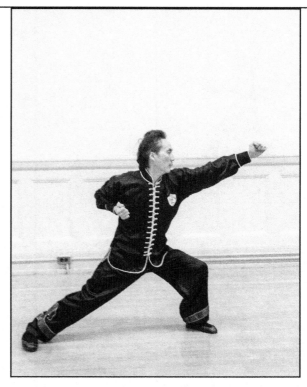

25) Right foot stamps. Right overhead block. Step forward with the left foot into a left bow stance. Left vertical punch.

Stamp the right foot and block upward with the right hand. Move the right hand in a clockwise motion as you block upward. Keep both hands clenched as fists. As you step forward into a left bow stance, strike forward with a left vertical fist.

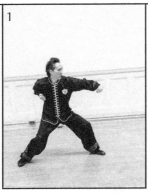

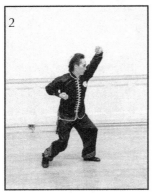

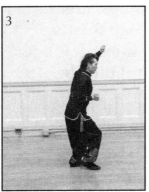

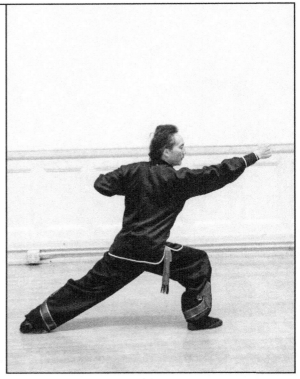

26) Left foot stamps. Left overhead block. Step forward with the right foot into a right bow stance. Right vertical punch.

Stamp the left foot and block upward with the left hand. Move the left hand in a counterclockwise motion as you block upward. Keep both hands clenched as fists. As you step forward into a right bow stance, strike forward with a right vertical fist

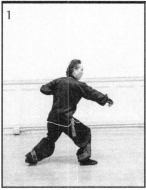

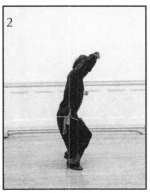

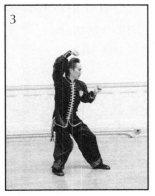

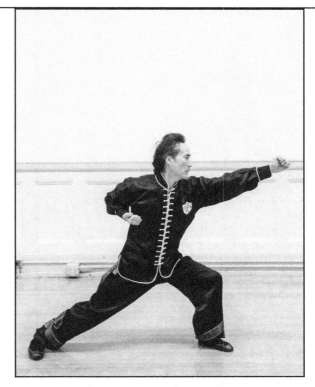

27) Right foot stamps. Right overhead block. Step forward with the left foot into a left bow stance. Left vertical punch.

Stamp the right foot and block upward with the right hand. Move the right hand in a clockwise motion as you block upward. Keep both hands clenched as fists. As you step forward into a left bow stance, strike forward with a left vertical fist.

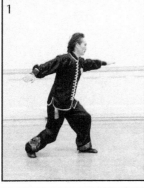

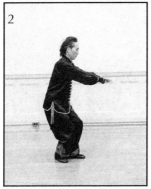

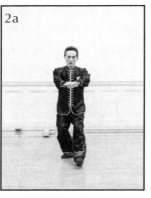

Side View

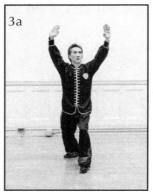

28) Back of right hand slaps left palm. Hands moving upward. Right foot stamps. Left heel.

Step forward and stamp the right foot on the ground. Step forward with the left foot. As you are moving forward, slap the back of the right hand into the palm of the left hand.

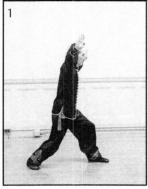

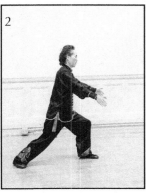

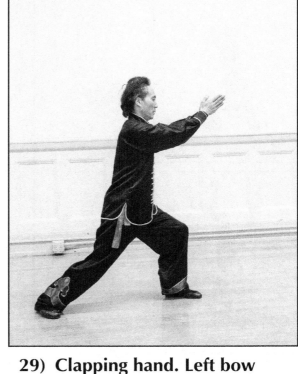

Side View

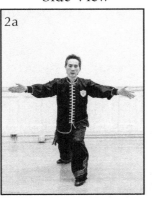

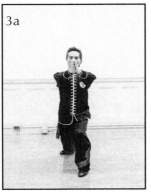

29) Clapping hand. Left bow stance (or transitory horse).

Continue the circular motion of the hands upward and then bring both hands down and around to clap the hands together. Most practitioners will clap their hands as they are moving upward. Temporarily, some might sit in a left bow stance but most practitioners will remain upright. This depends on how fast and how low in your stance you want to go. The photos portray a left bow stance but many will keep the weight somewhere between the right and left leg as the weight is being transferred from the right leg to the left leg. Either way is acceptable.

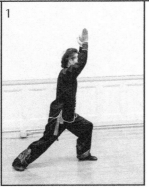

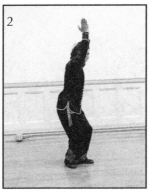

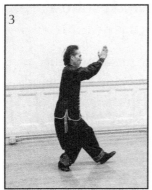

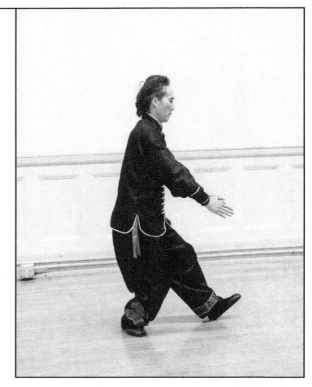

30) Clap downward.

Stamp the right foot on the ground and push the left foot forward (left foot on the heel) as you clap both hands downward. Both legs are slightly bent and more weight is on the right leg.

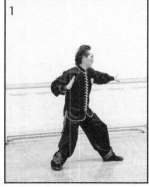

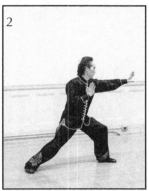

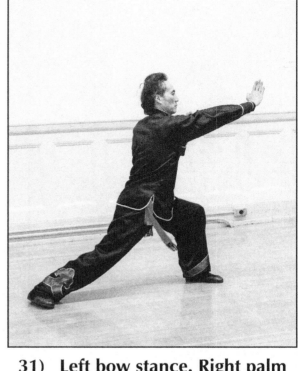

Side View

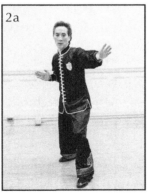

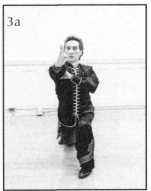

31) Left bow stance. Right palm thrust.

Finally, step forward with the left leg into a left bow stance and shoot the blade edge of the right hand forward (fingers pointing upward). The left hand blocks inward and retracts to the guard position along the right armpit. The left hand moves in a clockwise motion

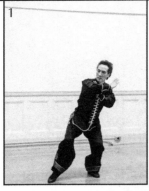

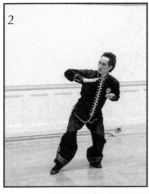

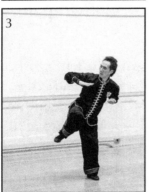

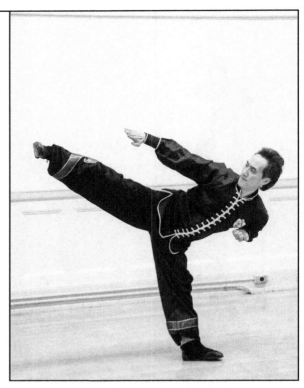

32) Turn to the right. Right side kick. Right upward clearing palm.

Turn to your right and kick outward in the opposite direction with the right leg. This is a right side kick and may be executed either high or low. Block upward and out with and open right hand. The fingertips of the right hand will point to your left. The left hand becomes a fist a fist (fist heart facing upward) and is held at the left side of your body.

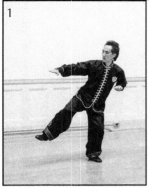

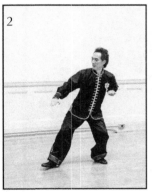

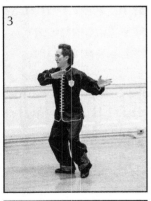

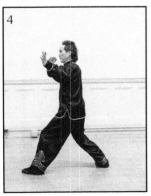

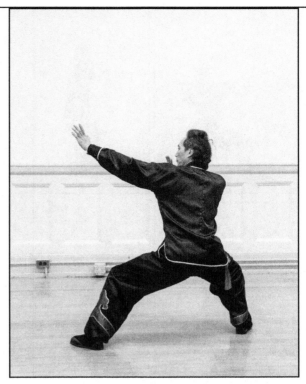

33) Right foot stamps. Left foot steps up. On guard position.

Step down with the right foot and bring the left foot forward. As you shift into the 4-6 stance with the weight mostly on the rear right leg, make a small clockwise motion with the right hand, and strike with a left open hand using a clockwise motion. The right hand held open near your face with the palm facing to the right side and the left arm is slightly bent with the left hand held at arm's length.

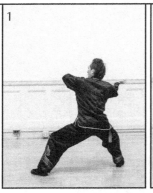

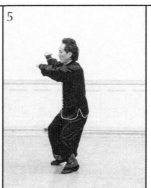

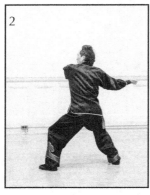

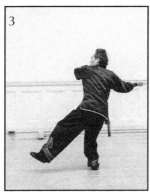

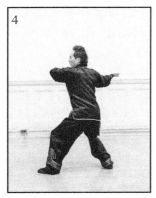

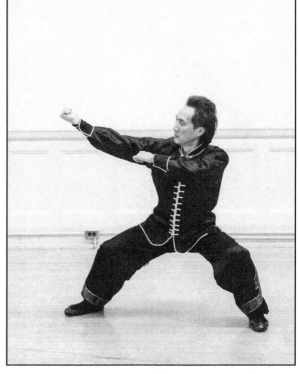

34) Left foot stamps. Right foot steps up. 4-6 stance (weight on the left leg). Right hammer fist.

Stamp the left foot and bring both hands back as fists with the left fist heart facing down and the right fist heart facing up. Then bring the right foot past the left into a 4-6 stance with the weight on the rear left leg. As you move forward, swing both arms forward and strike with a right hammer fist. The left fist heart remains facing downward. Your blow with the right hand is moving from the right side to the left.

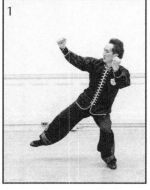

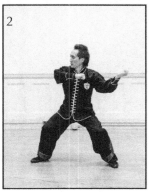

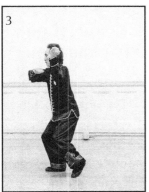

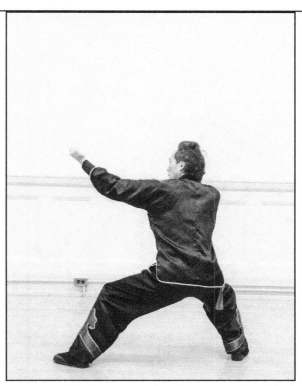

35) Right foot stamps. Left foot steps up. 4-6 stance (weight on the right leg). Left hammer fist.

Stamp the right foot and bring both hands back as fists with the right fist heart facing down and the left fist heart facing up. Then bring the left foot past the right into a 4-6 stance with the weight on the rear right leg. As you move forward, swing both arms forward and strike with a left hammer fist. The right fist heart remains facing downward. Your blow with the left hand is moving from the left side to the right. The right fist is held chambered at the right side of your body.

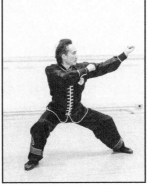

Back View

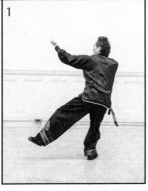

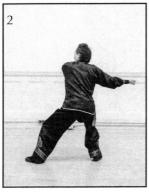

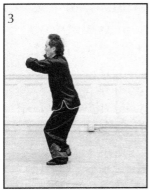

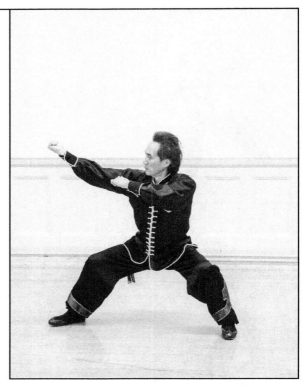

36) Left foot stamps. Right foot steps up. 4-6 stance (weight on the left leg). Right hammer fist.

Stamp the left foot and bring both hands back as fists with the left fist heart facing down and the right fist heart facing up. Then bring the right foot past the left into a 4-6 stance with the weight on the rear left leg. As you move forward, swing both arms forward and strike with a right hammer fist. The left fist heart remains facing downward. Your blow with the right hand is moving from the right side to the left.

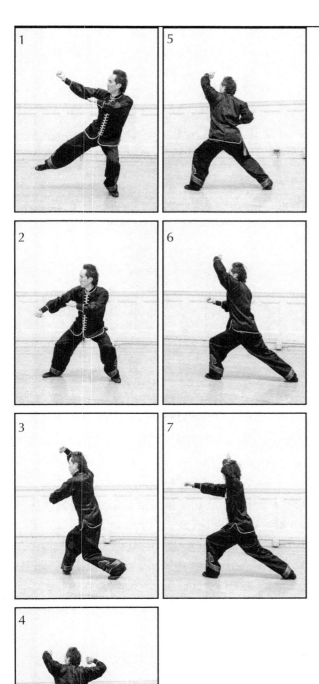

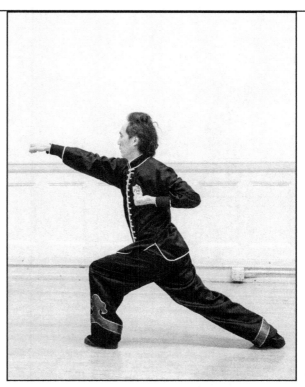

37) Right, left upward blocks. Right fist strike.

Stamp the right foot and step forward into a left bow stance. You may transition into this stance by first temporarily sitting in a right T-stance. Block up and outward (clockwise) with the right forearm, followed by a rising (counterclockwise) block of the left forearm. Finally, strike forward with a right horizontal fist. The left fist moves to the left side of your body with the fist heart of the left hand facing upward.

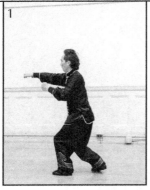

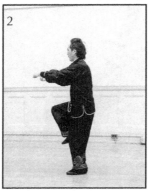

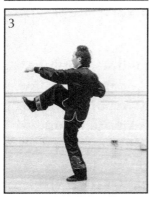

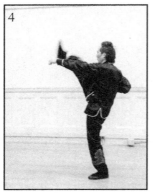

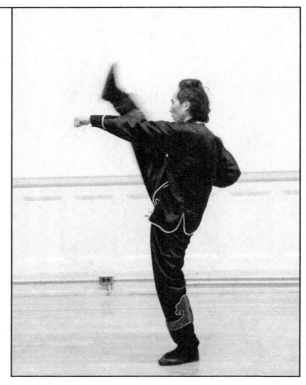

38. Left fist strike. Right toe kick.

Shift your weight on to your left leg and simultaneously, execute a high toe kick with the right foot while punching forward with a left horizontal fist. Do not let the weight on your hips extend too far forward. In other words, let the hips move forward but only slightly. This is done in anticipation of the next move. In other words, keep your weight back as you throw out your kick.

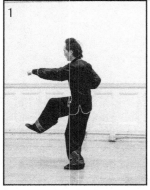

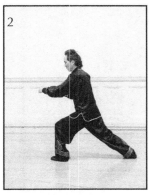

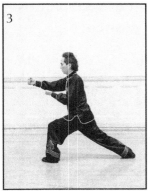

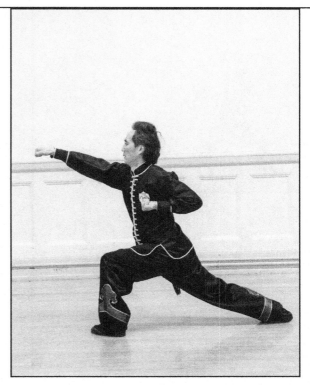

39. Retract the left fist. Right fist strike.

Retract the right leg and bring it back so that you sit in the same left bow stance as before the previous kick. As you bring the right leg back, strike forward with a right horizontal fist and bring the left fist back (palm up) to the left side of your body.

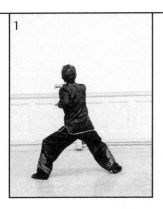

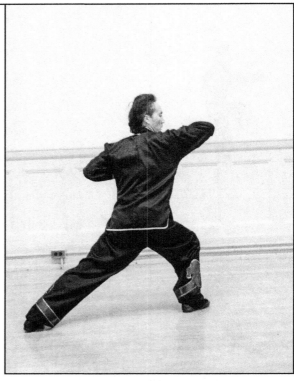

40. Turn to the right. Right elbow strike. Right bow stance.

Turn to your right and shift into a right bow stance. Strike with the right elbow as your torso turns to the right side. This is a sideways elbow strike. You are striking in the opposite direction of where you previously faced. Both hands are held as closed fists.

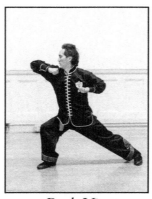

Back View

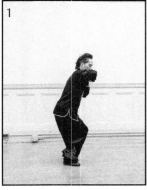

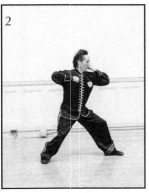

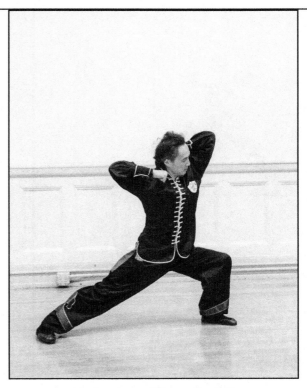

41. Step forward in a left bow stance. Rising elbow strike.

Step forward with the left foot into a left bow stance. While moving forward, strike upward with the left elbow. The left fist ends near your left ear with the fist heart facing down. The right fist (palm down) remains facing downward and is now near your right cheek.

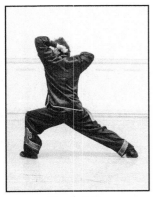

Back View

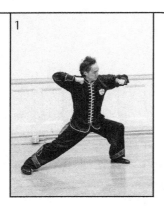

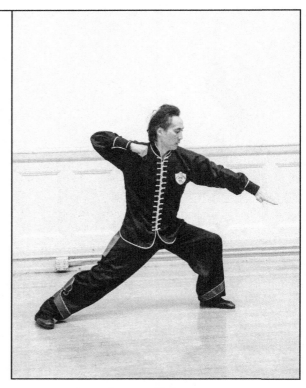

42. Left palm strike.

Strike down with the left hand. The palm of the left hand will face the ground and the fingertips will point to your right. The left hand will make a slight clockwise downward arc.

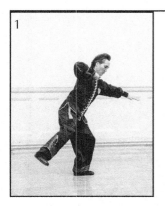

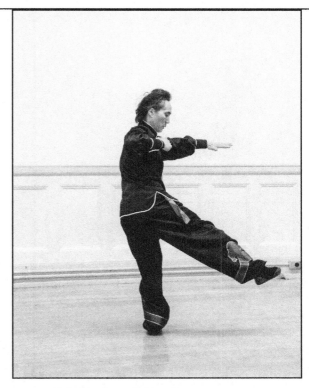

43. Right hooking leg.

Move the right leg in a counterclockwise motion and hook with the right instep.

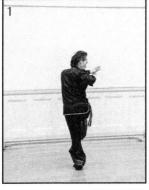

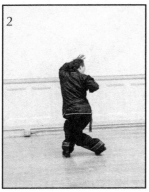

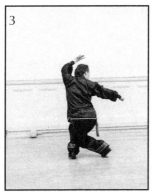

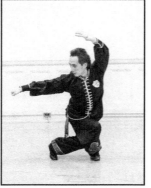

Back View

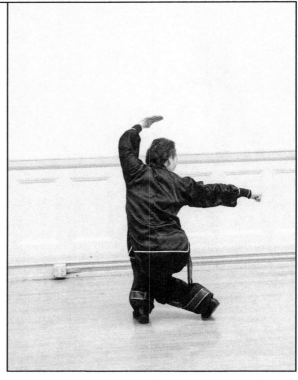

44. Left clears upward. Right fist strike.

Swing the right foot all the way around to the left side so you end in a right T-stance. Then block upward with the left hand using a counterclockwise motion. Open the left hand as you block upward. The left palm will face to the sky. The right hand will move in a counterclockwise motion as you pull it back and then strike down with a right horizontal fist.

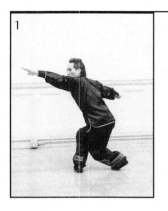

1

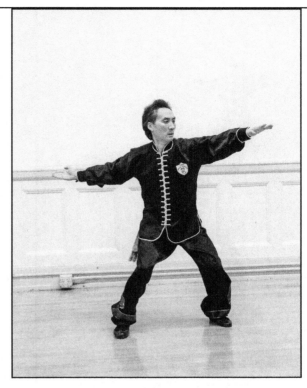

45. Turn the body. Left bow stance. Left slashing palm.

Twist your body to the left and clear with the left hand (palm facing downward). Your left hand moves in a counterclockwise motion. You may temporarily sit in a left bow stance and this depends on how fast you withdraw your left leg to bring it around.

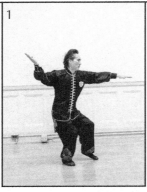

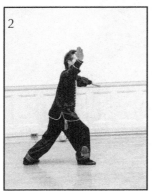

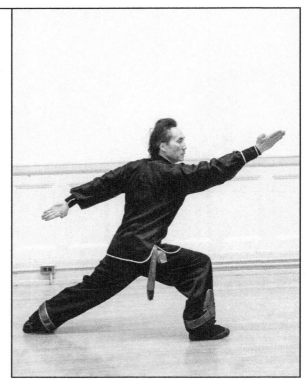

46. Left pulling hand. Right bow stance. Right chopping palm.

Completely withdraw the left leg past the right leg and chop with the right hand as you shift into a right bow stance. The right palm may face up and be slightly turned to the left side, i.e. the right palm may strike downward at a 45 degree angle. The left hand is now behind you with the palm facing down and to the back.

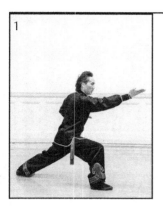

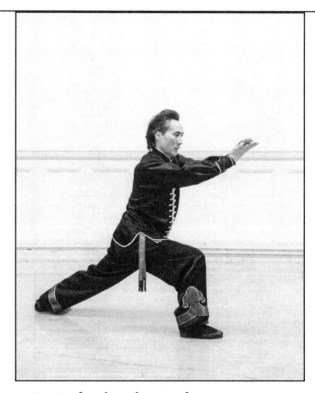

47. Left piercing palm.

Finally, bring the right foot back alongside the left foot and shoot the left hand forward (palm up) so that it rests in the palm of the right hand.

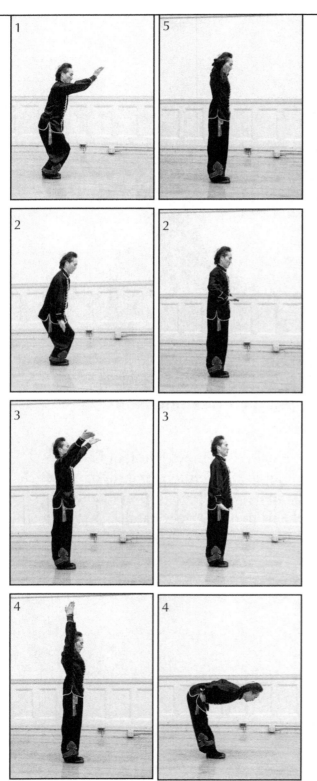

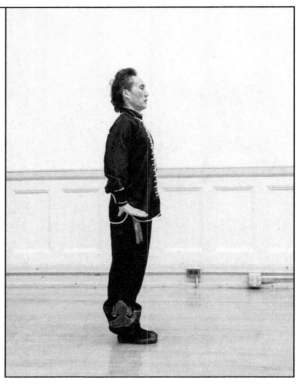

48) Withdraw and bow. The set is complete.

Then swing both hands down, then up, and down once more. Bow. The set has now been completed.

Siu Wan Kuen - Applications

The applications are shown in a way that is similar to the moves in the form. It was done in this way so that one may more clearly see the relation of the move in the form to the application. Of course, in actual self-defense scenarios, do not worry about how the move looks. Be practical and realistic.

Application Moves 1-4

You are aimlessly daydreaming your life away, when…. all of a sudden…someone tries to grab you around the neck! Break his grip by pushing his hands off you. Then strike him in the chest with both fists. Of course, if he grabs you with one hand, you may brush his hand off of you by using only one of your hands. Then strike him quickly with that same hand, or the other hand as appropriate.

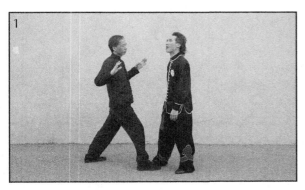

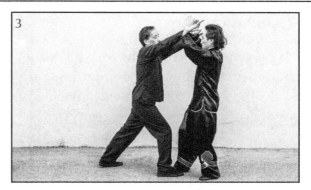

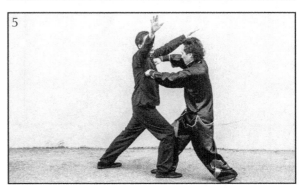

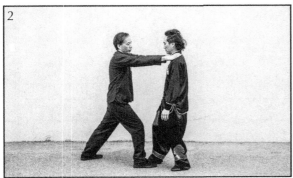

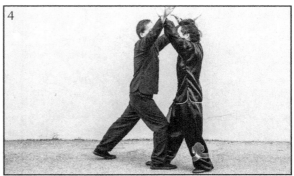

Application Moves 5-6

If he swings down at you with his left hand, use an 'X-block' upward using both arms. Then strike him in the stomach with your left fist.

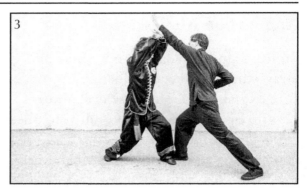

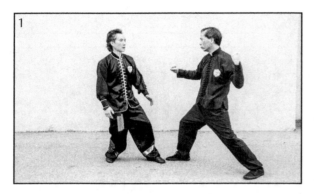

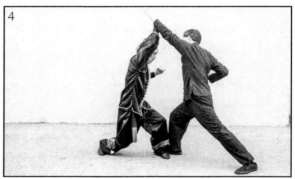

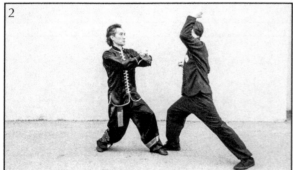

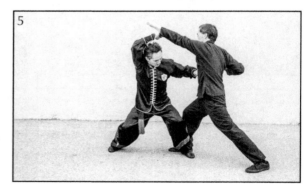

Application Move 7

If he kicks you with his right foot, block outward with your left forearm. Strike him in the groin with your right fist. Then sing the words, "Hello, is it me you're looking for?"

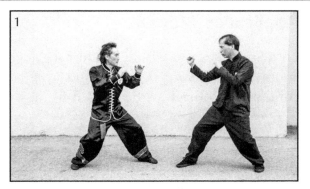

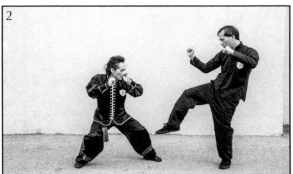

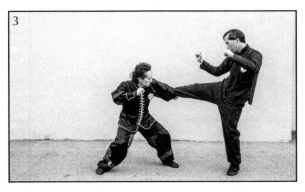

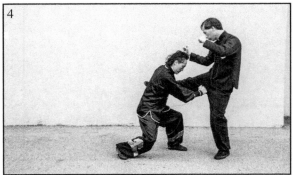

Application Move 8

If he punches you with his right fist, block it upward with your right arm and strike him in the stomach with your left fist.

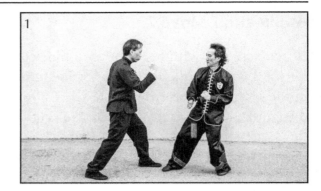

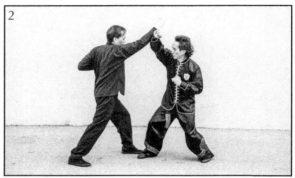

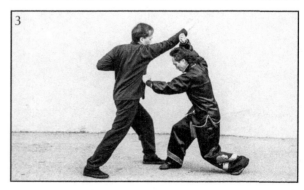

Application Move 9

As he punches you with his left arm, grab hold of his arm, twist it and force him down.

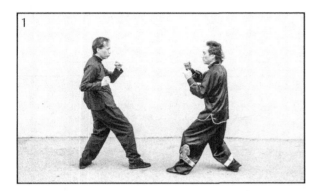

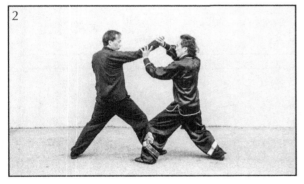

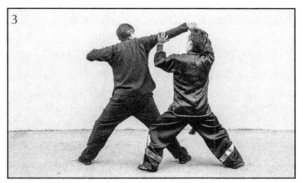

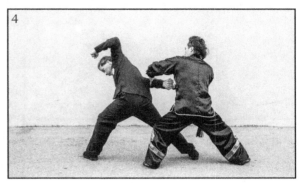

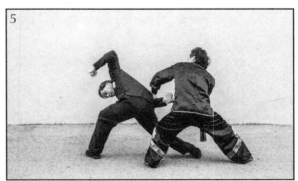

Application Move 9 Alternate

Alternatively, as he punches you with his left arm, grab his arm, twist it down and then up. This will also force his body down.

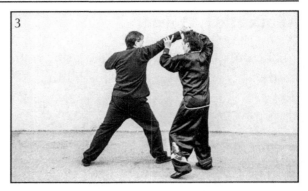

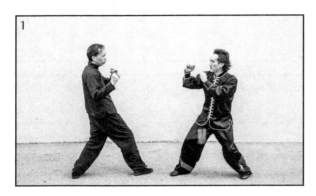

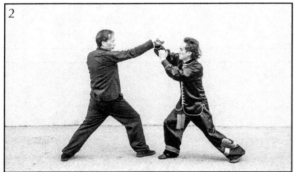

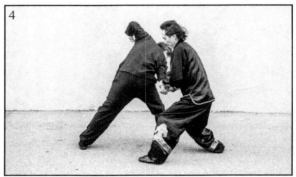

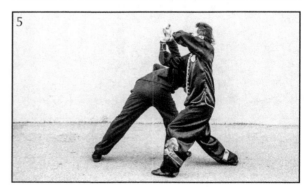

Application Moves 10 – 11

Movement #10 can be seen as a transition move and also may be interpreted as a knee strike to the opponent's midsection or thigh region. This application is not pictured here. Only the application with the hands is shown.

If he punches you with his right arm, grab his arm and lift it up. Then step in and punch him with both fists to drive him back.

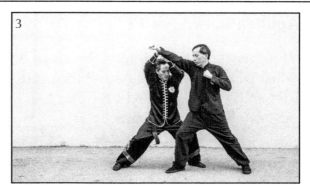

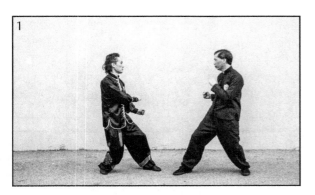

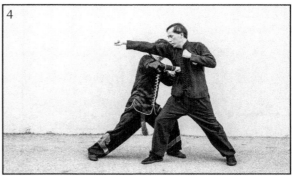

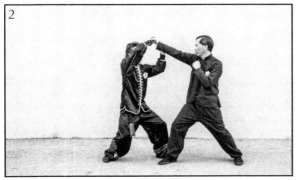

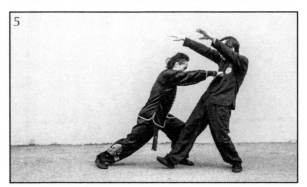

Application Move 12

If he punches you with his right arm, grab it first with your right hand and then your left hand. Follow this up by kneeing him in the side with your left knee.

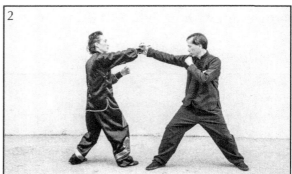

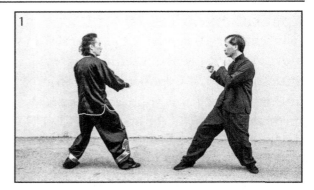

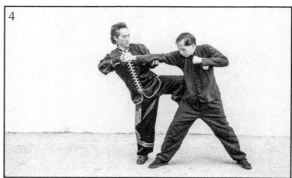

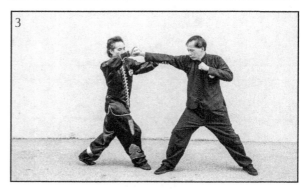

Application Move 12: Alternate

As he kicks you with his right foot, parry it upward and to the side using your left instep.

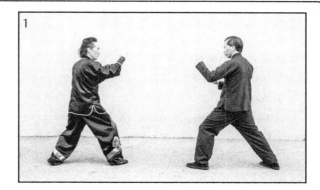

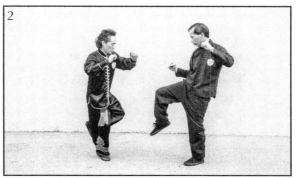

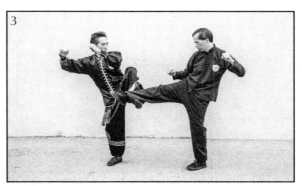

Application Moves 13-14

If he punches you with his left hand, grab it with your left hand and smash down on his elbow with your right forearm. Follow this up by punching him in the face with your fist(s).

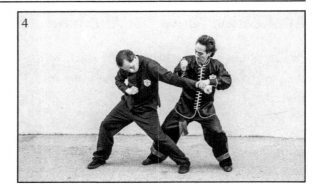

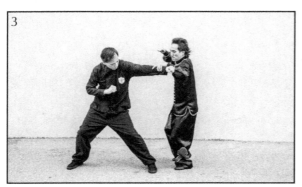

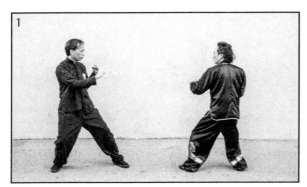

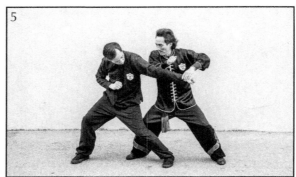

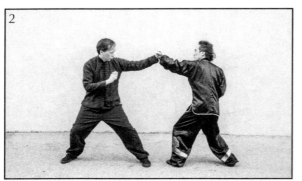

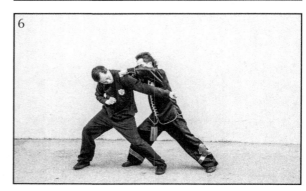

Application Moves 15-16

Initiate the attack with a left elbow strike. As he attempt to block it with his right arm, lift up his arm with your left hand and strike him with your right hand.

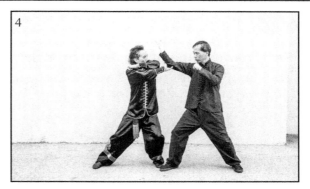

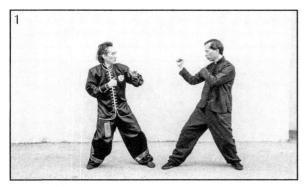

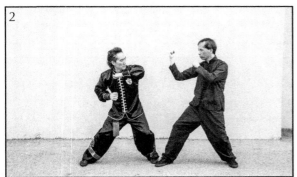

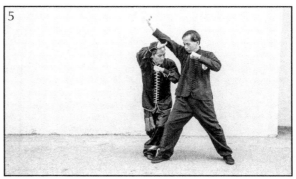

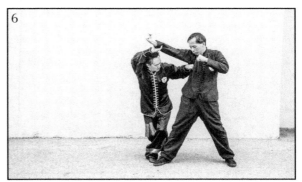

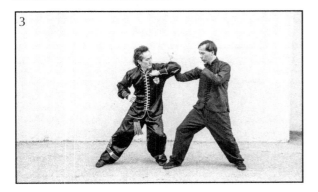

Application Move 17

As he moves to punch you with his right fist, grab his right arm with your right hand and then punch down at his head with your left hand.

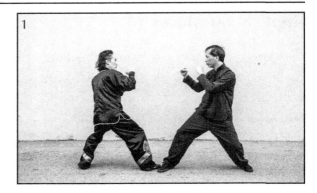

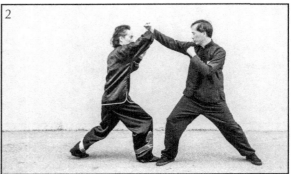

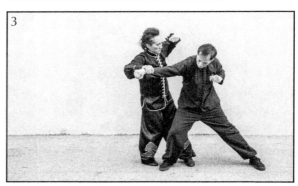

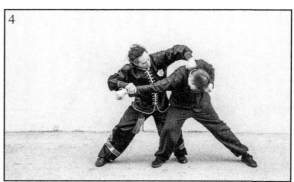

Application Move 18

If he strikes down at you with his right arm, block upward with your left arm and strike him under the chin with your left fist.

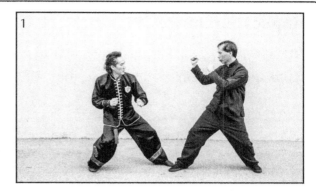

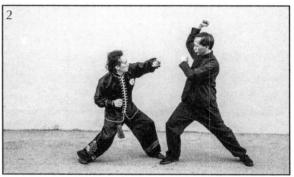

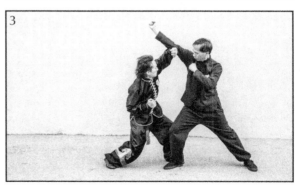

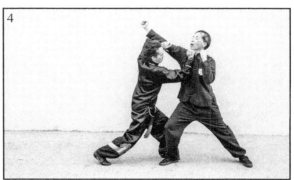

Application Move 19

Block his left punch down with your left hand and kick him with your left foot.

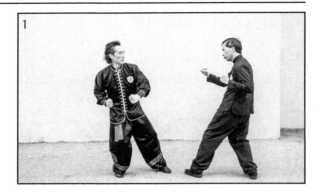

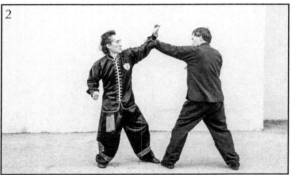

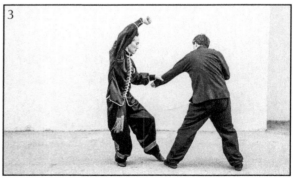

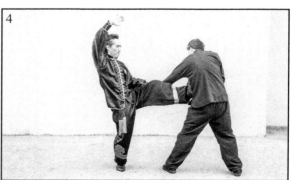

Application Move 20

Or initiate a right kick, and when the opponent moves to block it, strike down at him with a right backfist.

When moves are done simultaneously, one may be offense, the other defense, or vice-versa.

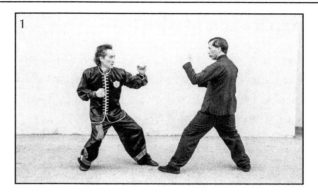

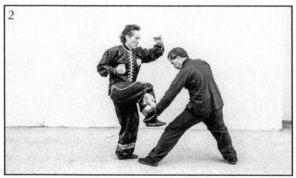

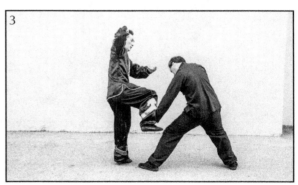

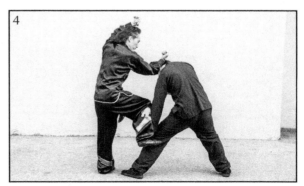

Application Move 21

As he moves in to strike you with his right fist, lean back, turn around to take away his target, block his strike with your left hand and then kick him with a left side kick.

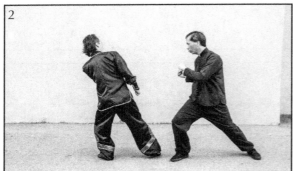

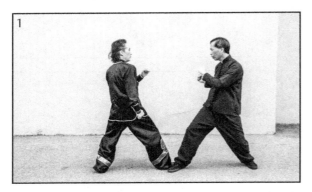

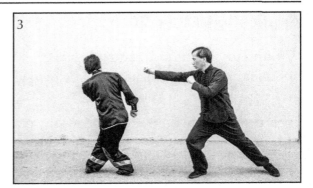

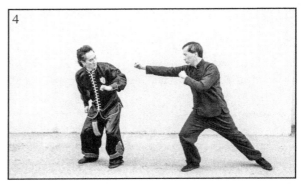

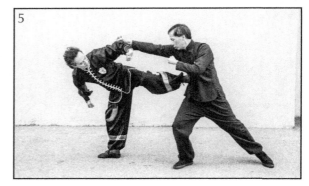

Application Move 22

Block his left punch down with your left forearm. Twist your body and strike him with your right fist.

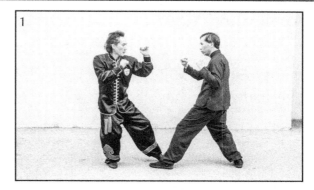

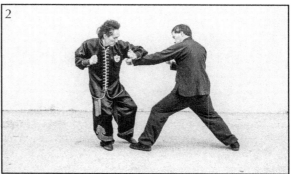

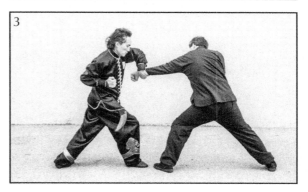

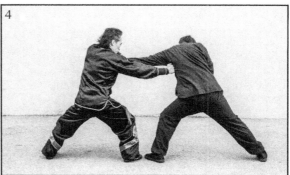

Application Move 23

This is the same move but on the other side. Block down with your right and punch him with your left hand.

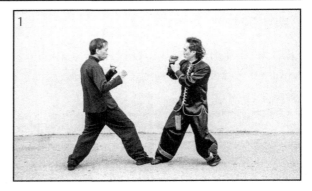

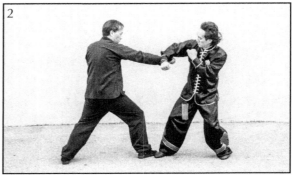

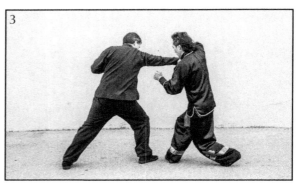

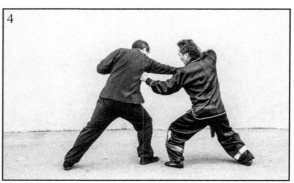

Application Move 24

As he punches you with his left hand, block his strike, down and to the side with your left hand. Strike him with your right hand and twist your waist to get more power into your blow.

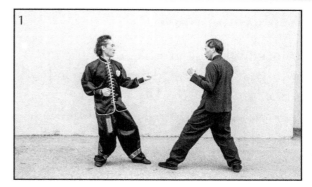

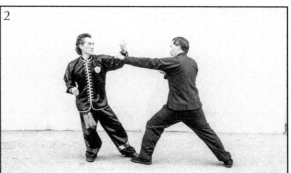

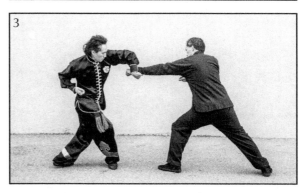

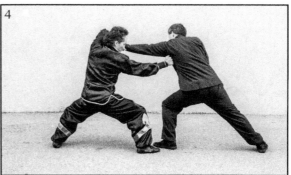

Application Move 25

Block his left hand strike by lifting up with your right arm. Then step in and strike him with your left fist.

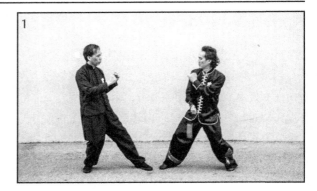

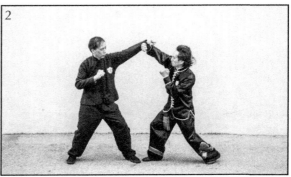

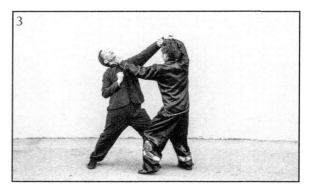

Application Move 26

This is the same move but on the other side.

Block upward with your left arm, then strike him with your right fist.

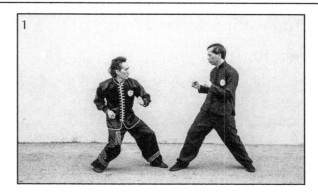

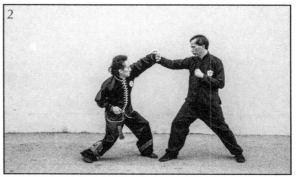

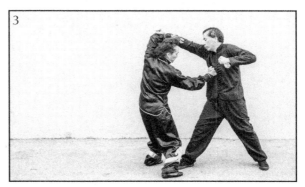

Application Move 27

Block his left arm strike with your right arm, then move in and strike him with your left fist.

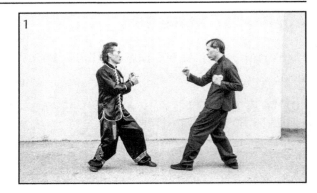

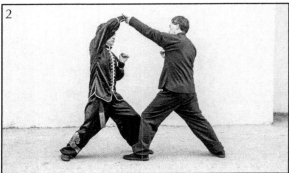

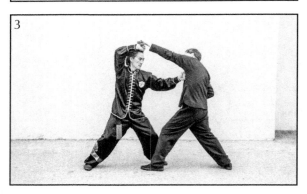

Application Moves 28-29-30-31

You are looking away and he catches you unawares. You feel his hands around your neck. Raise both of hands upward to break his grip. Then after his grip has been broken, slap both of his ears with the palms of your hands. Then do it again (with even more force). Finally, strike him in the neck with the blade edge of your right hand. This is the cure for a nefarious man with ill-intent bent on strangling you. Isn't it nice to have the good guys win every once in a while?

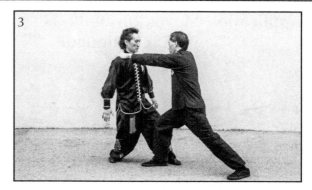

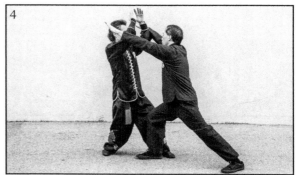

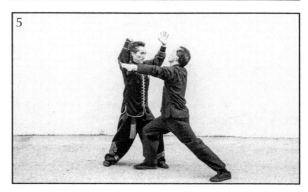

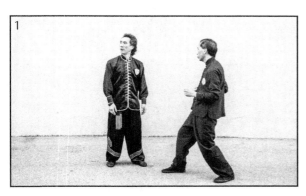

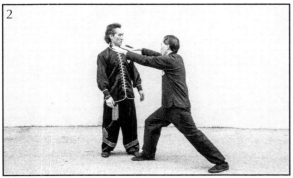

Continued on next page

Application Moves 28-29-30-31
(Continued)

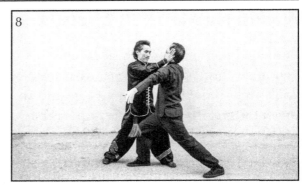

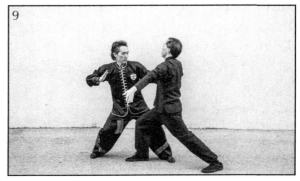

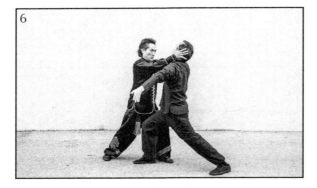

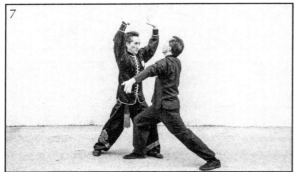

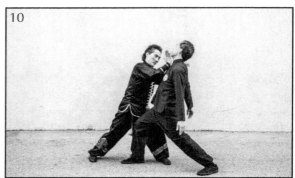

Application Move 32

You are looking away. At the last moment, you see someone behind you attempting to strike you with a right hammer blow. Turn quickly, block upward with your right arm and then give him a strong side kick with your right leg. Try and be aware of your surroundings at all times, and remember, protect that smart-phone!

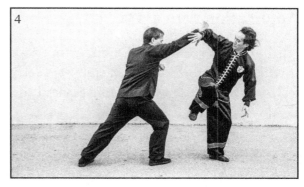

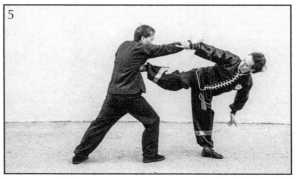

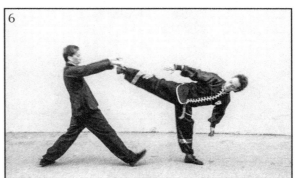

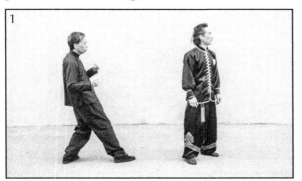

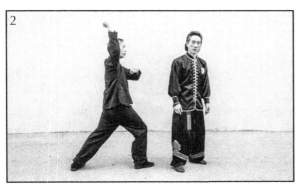

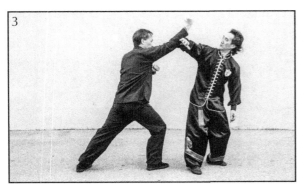

Application Move 33

As he strikes you with his right arm, parry it with your right arm. Then step your left leg forward and slap him in the back of his head with your left palm.

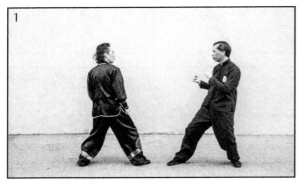

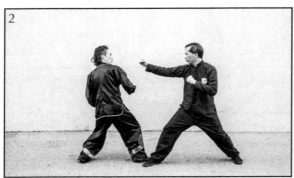

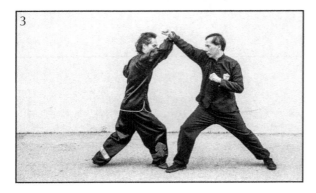

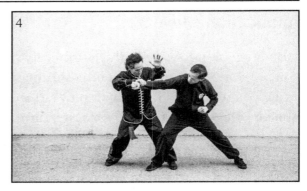

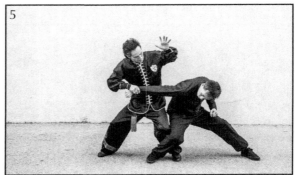

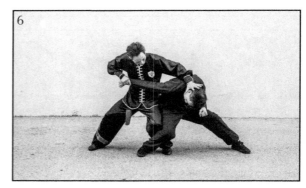

Application Move 34

As he punches you with his left arm, parry it with your own left arm. Then jam your right knee into the back of his left leg to break his balance. Strike him in the neck or the back of his head with a right hammer fist.

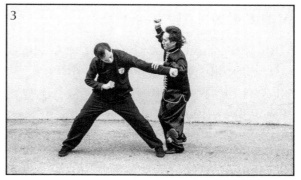

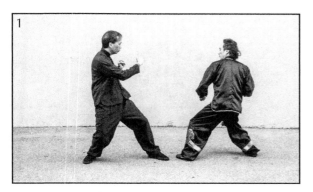

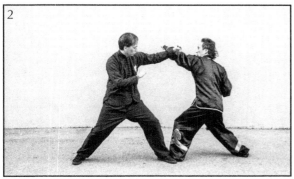

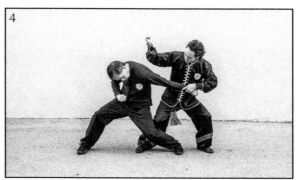

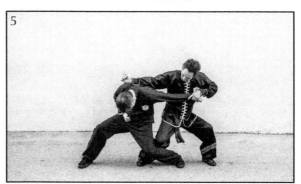

Application Move 35

This is the same move but on the other side. He grabs your right wrist with his right hand. Bend your right arm, step in and smash him in the back with your left forearm. Although the move is the same in the set, the same move may be used to react to different scenarios.

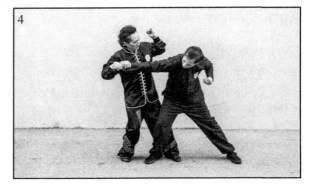

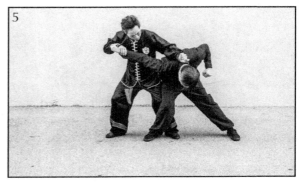

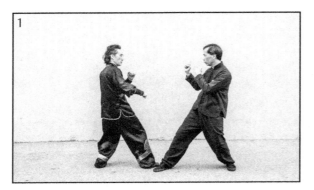

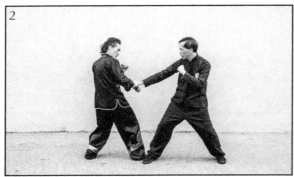

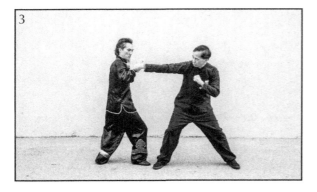

Move 36 has the same application as move #35.

Application Move 37

Block his right fist strike upward with your right forearm. Block his left fist strike with your left forearm. Drive in and punch him with your right fist.

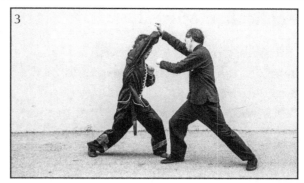

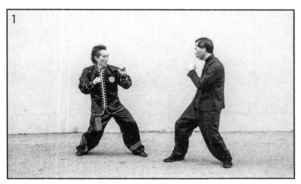

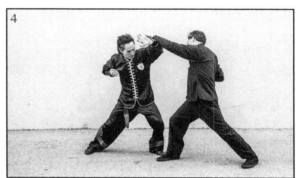

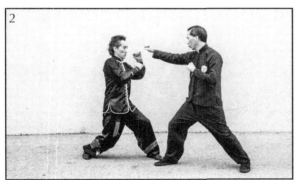

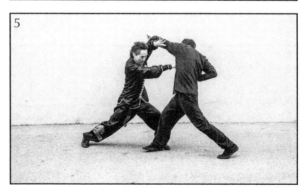

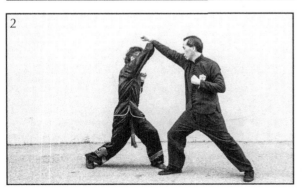

Application Move 38

He grabs your right wrist with his left hand. Raise your right forearm and kick him with your right foot. If he tries to block your right kick, punch him in the face with your left hand. What you do depends on how he reacts and what he does. It's actually not easy to do two strikes at one time.

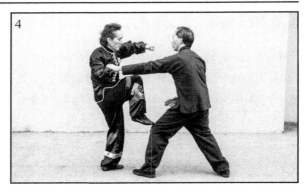

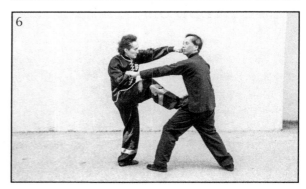

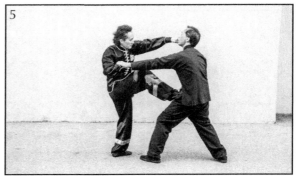

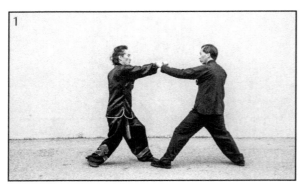

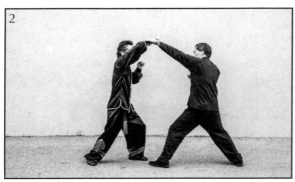

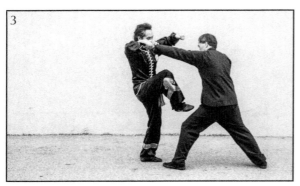

Application Move 39

If he grabs your left wrist with his right
hand to shake you down, the solution
is simple, punch him in the face with
your free right hand. React quickly and
immediately, and punch with force. Simple
is always good.

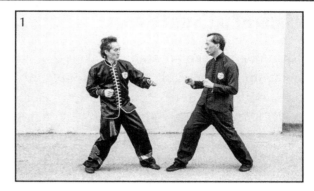

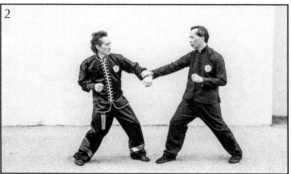

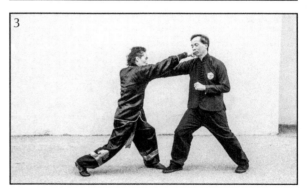

Application Moves 40-41

Bridging the gap with an initial elbow strike might not work. In this example, it is done with the intent of making him react. As he reacts to your right elbow strike with his right hand, step forward and strike him using your left elbow.

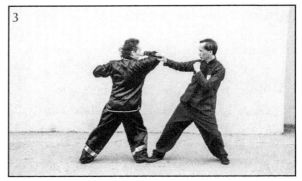

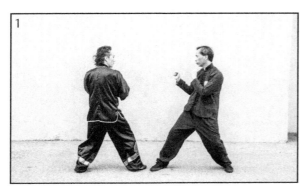

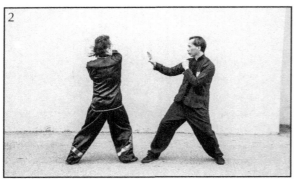

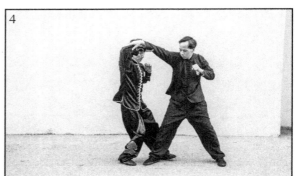

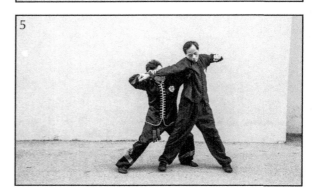

Application Moves 42-43-44

Force him to react by moving your hand downward as a left palm strike. As he parries it with his left arm, use a right hook kick and kick his left leg out from under him. Unbalance him. Then, follow through and strike him in the back with your right fist.

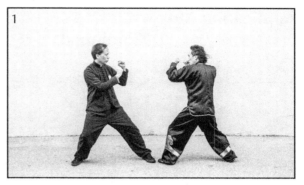

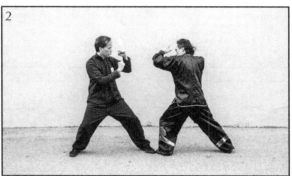

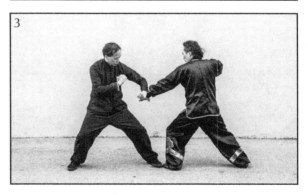

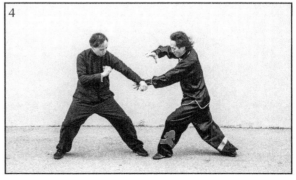

Continued on next page

Application Moves 42-43-44
(Continued)

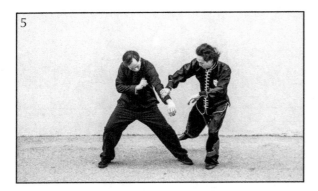

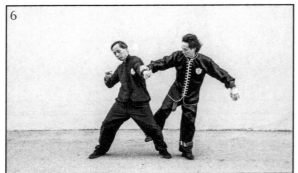

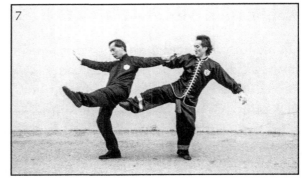

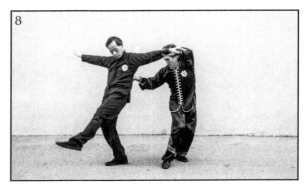

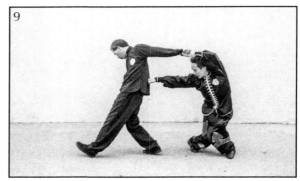

Application Moves 45-46

As he reaches out to grab you with his left hand, turn around to take away his intended target. Yank him downward with your left hand and chop him in the back of his neck with the blade edge of your right hand. Chop him hard at the base of his neck. Verbal deflection does not always work against a hard-core bully. This might.

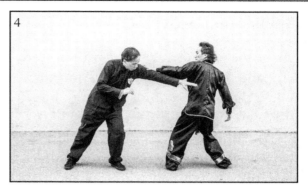

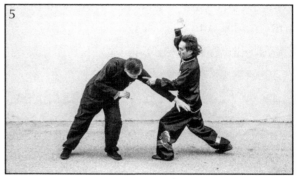

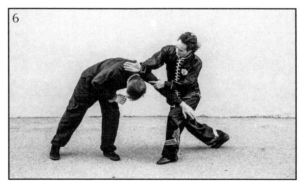

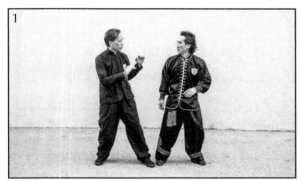

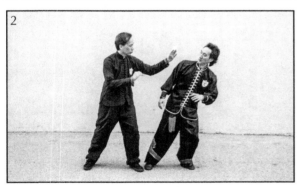

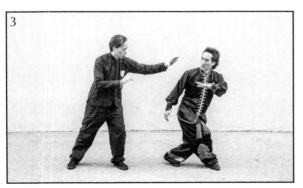

Application Moves 47

As he grabs your right wrist with his left hand, turn your right hand over to relieve the pressure of his grip or to break or loosen his grip. Then spear him in the throat with the fingertips of your left hand. If you apply this move successfully, the bully will typically adopt a more conciliatory tone... that is... if he still has a tone remaining.

And that, my friends, is the end of the applications section.

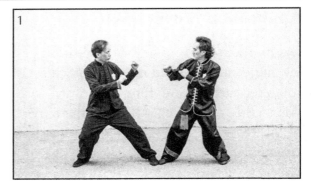

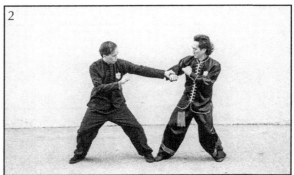

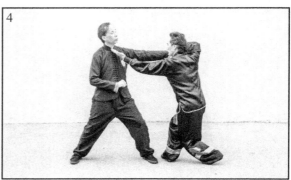

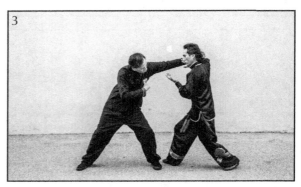

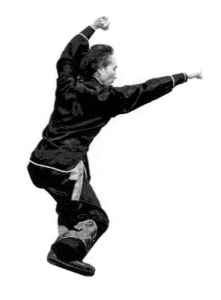

APPENDIX A: SIDE VIEW OF COMPLETE SET

(The following pictures are ordered from up to down, and then left to right.)

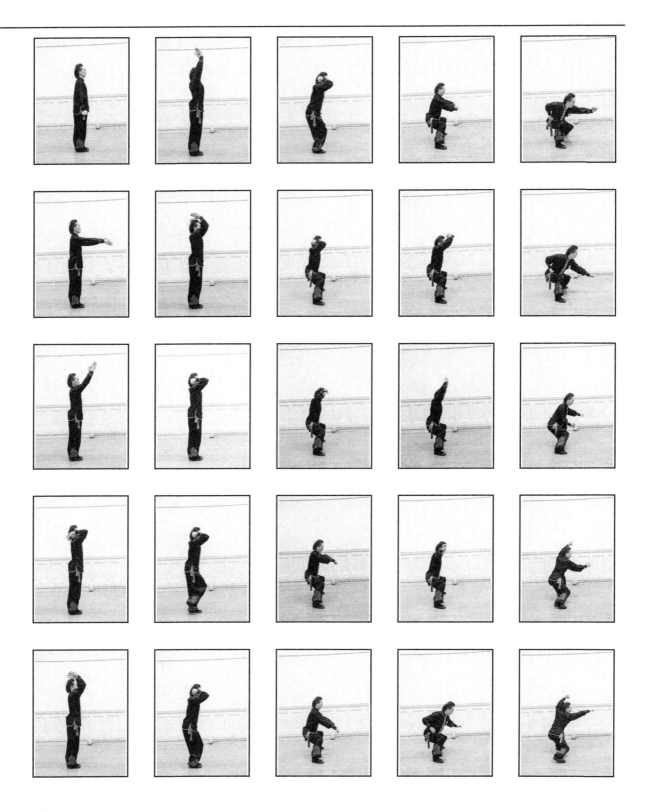

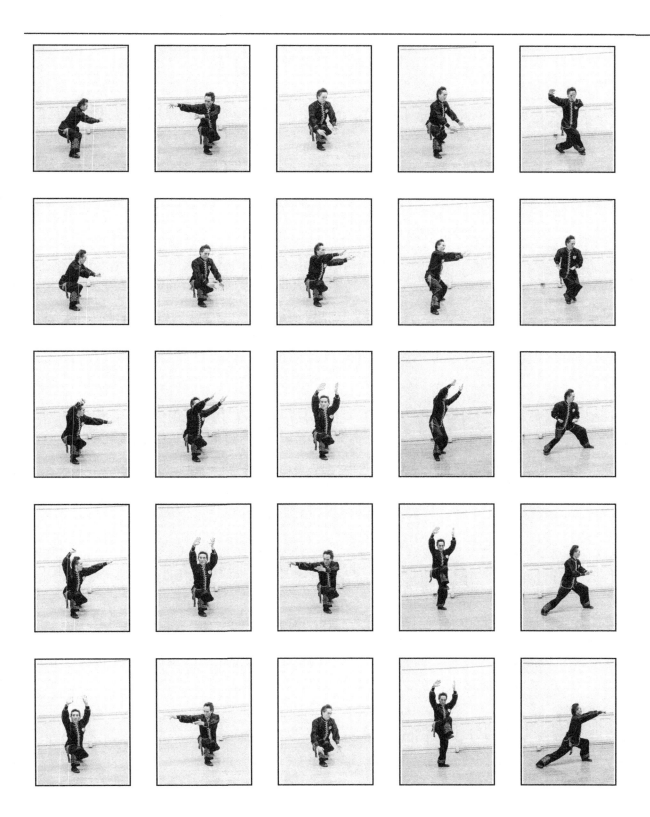

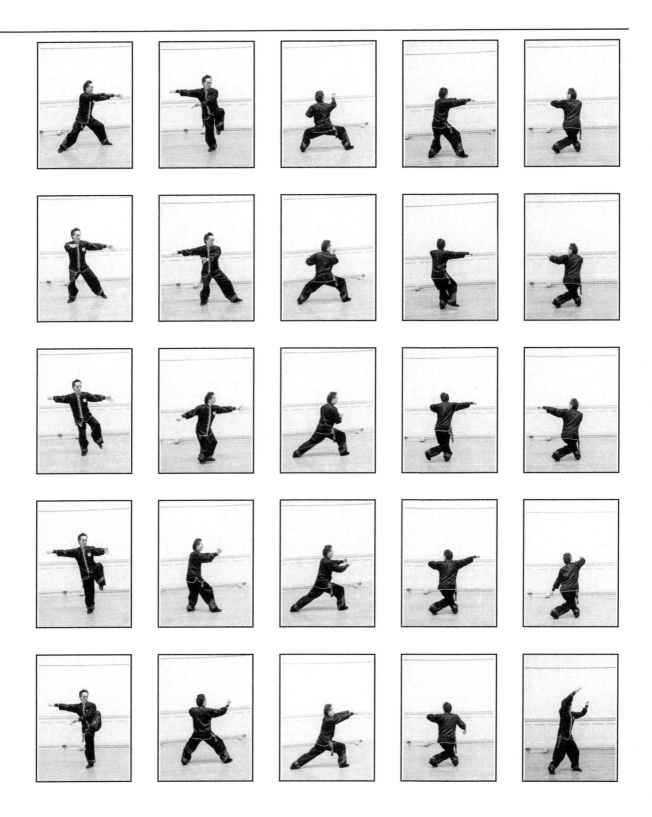

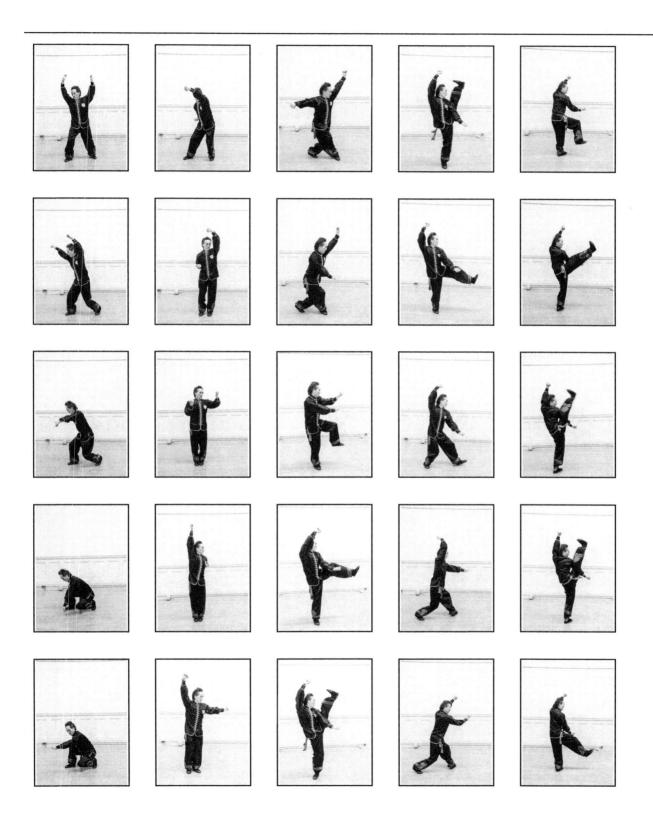

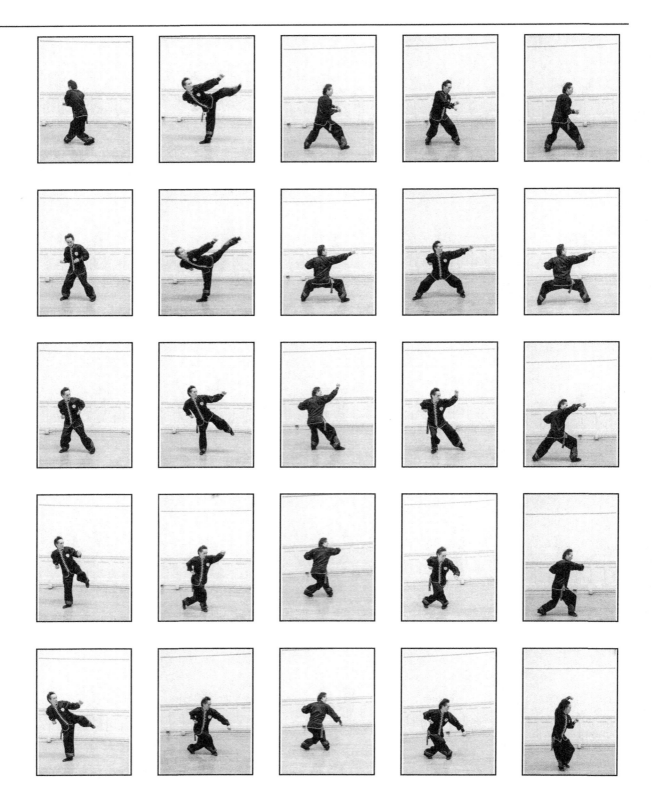

124

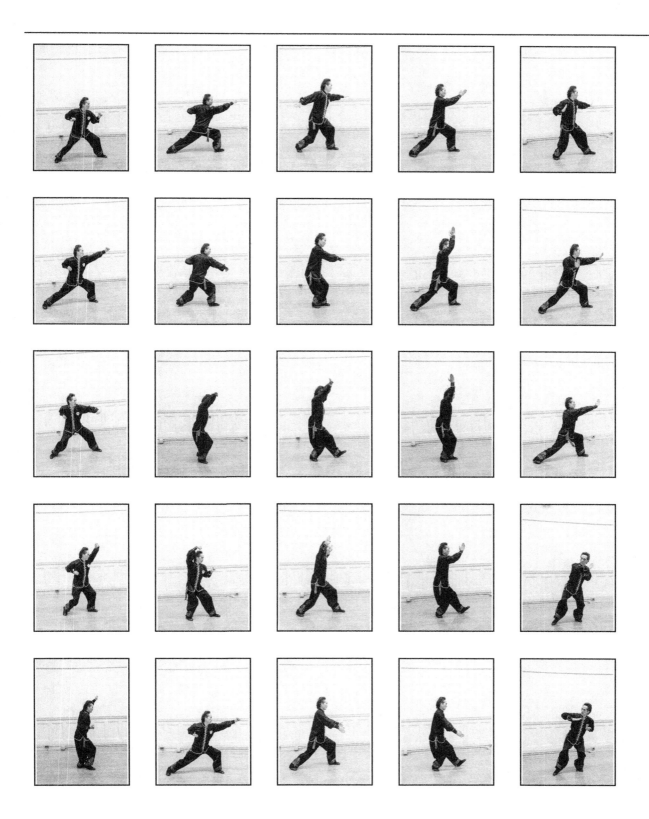

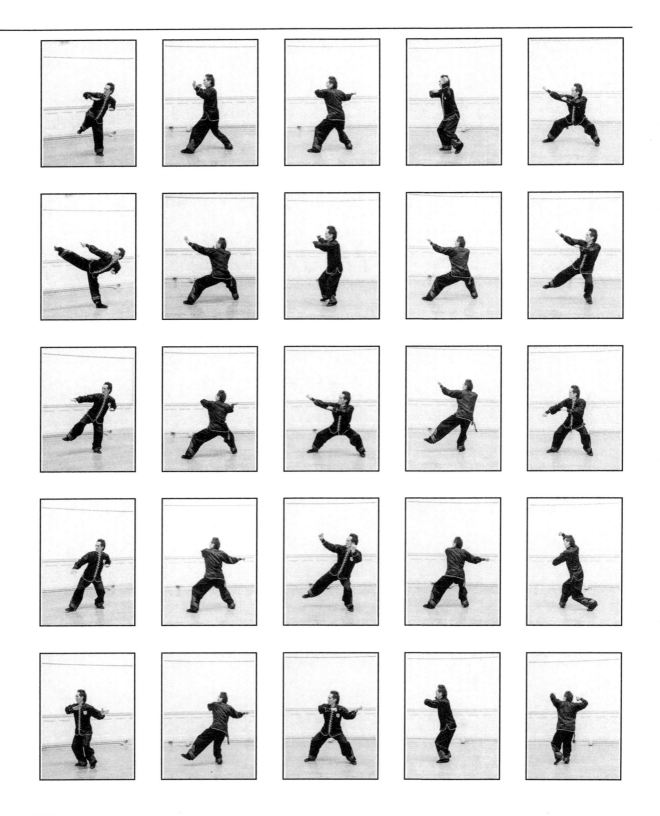

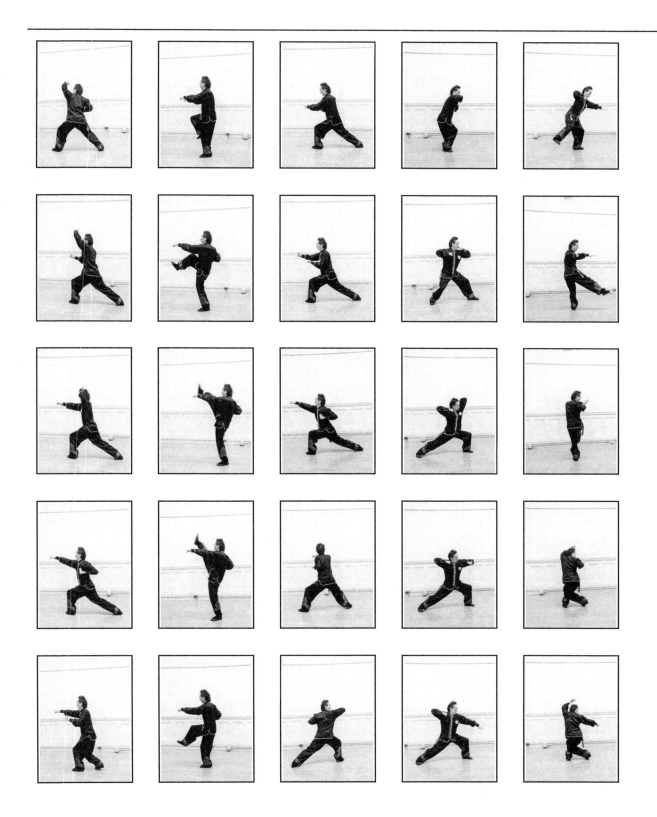

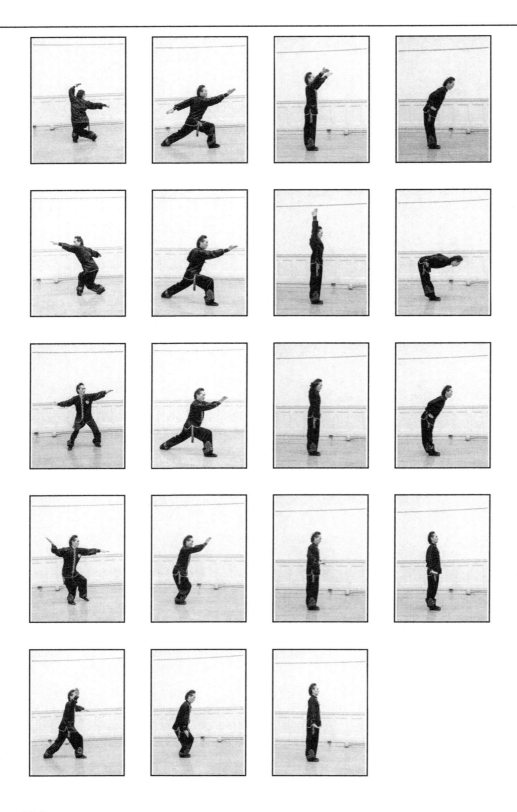

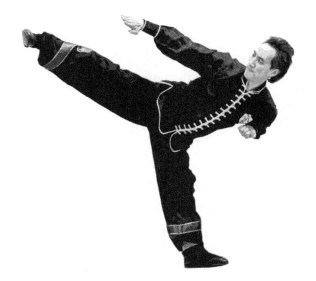

APPENDIX B: SHORT NAMES FOR SET

1) Listen for Buddha. Thrust palms to the sky.

2) Pull hands down to the ears and form fists with both hands.

3) Stamp the right foot. Horse stance.

4) Double fists strike downward.

5) "X" (Cross) block above the head.

6) Left punch. Twisted stance.

7) Right punch. Strike straight ahead. Twisted stance. Right knee forward.

8) Left punch. Strike straight ahead. Twisted stance. Left knee forward.

9) Double (clockwise) circular hands. Three times. Move hands like the wind. Create a whirlwind with the hands.

10) Raise the right leg. Raise both hands high.

11) Double dragons (horizontal) fist strike. Double charging fists. Clockwise motion. Left bow stance.

12) Step back. Crane stance. Left leg raised. Left palm faces the sky.

13) Left grabbing hand. Left foot steps down into a horse stance. Right arm (forearm or fist) breaks the opponent's arm.

14) Double dragon (horizontal) fists. Strike to the right. Right bow stance.

15) Step back into left T-stance. Left battering elbow strike.

16) Right hand to the guard position. Left (horizontal) punch.

17) Turn to the right. Reach to the sky. Right grabbing hand. Left fist follows. Smash down to the ground. Crouching stance.

18) Right punch to the sky. Stand up straight.

19) Right hand blocks up. Left backfist strikes down. Left heel kick.

20) Left hand blocks up. Right backfist strikes down. Right heel kick.

21) Turn around. Left side kick. Left vertical punch.

22) Left hand blocks down. Right vertical fist. Sit in a horse stance.

23) Right hand blocks down. Left vertical fist. Sit in a horse stance.

24) Left hand blocks down. Right vertical fist. Sit in a horse stance.

25) Right foot stamps. Right overhead block. Step forward with the left foot into a left bow stance. Left vertical punch.

26) Left foot stamps. Left overhead block. Step forward with the right foot into a right bow stance. Right vertical punch.

27) Right foot stamps. Right overhead block. Step forward with the left foot into a left bow stance. Left vertical punch.

28) Back of right hand slaps left palm. Hands moving upward. Right foot stamps. Left heel.

29) Clapping hand. Left bow stance (or transitory horse).

30) Clap downward.

31) Left bow stance. Right palm thrust.

32) Turn to the right. Right side kick. Right upward clearing palm.

33) Right foot stamps. Left foot steps up. On guard position.

34) Left foot stamps. Right foot steps up. 4-6 stance (weight on the left leg). Right hammer fist.

35) Right foot stamps. Left foot steps up. 4-6 stance (weight on the right leg). Left hammer fist.

36) Left foot stamps. Right foot steps up. 4-6 stance (weight on the left leg). Right hammer fist.

37) Right, left upward blocks. Right fist strike.

38) Left fist strike. Right toe kick.

39) Retract the left fist. Right fist strike.

40) Turn to the right. Right elbow strike. Right bow stance.

41) Step forward in a left bow stance. Rising elbow strike.

42) Left palm strike.

43) Right hooking leg.

44) Left clears upward. Right fist strike.

45) Turn the body. Left bow stance. Left slashing palm.

46) Left pulling hand. Right bow stance. Right chopping palm.

47) Left piercing palm.

48) Withdraw and bow. The set is complete.

Acknowledgements

I'd like to thank Mr. Clint Boerner, the six foot three inch Scandinavian / Neanderthal warrior, for helping me design and assemble this book. I had kept this book on the back-burner (Boerner?) for far too long. I know nothing of his desktop publishing skills and my capacity was limited to that of "Chance the Gardener." "I was there," and "I like to watch," is all I can say. My little ideas and his big hands made this medium-size book come alive.

As before, and for all my previous books, I'd like to thank Phillip Wong for taking the photos. My timing need not be perfect, but his certainly does. He truly captures the moment.

I'd also like to thank Mr. Jeffrey Wing for helping in the applications section. Although he helped in the applications part, he is certainly no "dummy" and in fact, he is a licensed endodontist, and, needless to say, one way or another, he will get to the root of your dental problems. He's a tough guy and a better actor.

Ms. Fan Ching Kuo (strange initials really) also helped with the calligraphy. I helped but she maintains it was a stroke... of luck! A few strokes actually but she deserves the major credit for the calligraphy.

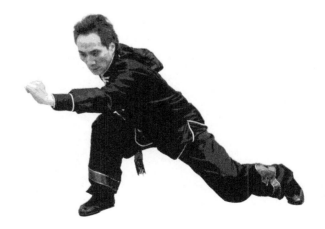

Printed in Great Britain
by Amazon

25752082R00077